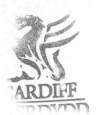

Having
Your Baby
THROUGH
Egg Donation

Having Your Baby

THROUGH

Egg Donation

Second Edition

Ellen Sarasohn Glazer
and Evelina Weidman Sterling

Jessica Kingsley *Publishers*
London and Philadelphia

618.178
GLA

First published in 2005 by Perspectives Press, Indianapolis, USA

This second edition published in 2013
by Jessica Kingsley Publishers
116 Pentonville Road
London N1 9JB, UK
and
400 Market Street, Suite 400
Philadelphia, PA 19106, USA

www.jkp.com

Library of Congress Cataloging in Publication Data
Glazer, Ellen Sarasohn.
  Having your baby through egg donation / Ellen Sarasohn Glazer
and Evelina Weidman Sterling. -- Second edition.
     pages cm
  Includes bibliographical references and index.
  ISBN 978-1-84905-901-5 (alk. paper)
 1. Human reproductive technology--Popular works. 2. Ovum--Transplantation.
3. Infertility--Psychological aspects. I. Sterling, Evelina Weidman, 1970- II. Title.
  RG133.5.G56 2013
  618.1'7806--dc23
                            2012049213

British Library Cataloguing in Publication Data
A CIP catalogue record for this book is available from the British Library

ISBN 978 1 84905 901 5
eISBN 978 0 85700 652 3

Printed and bound in Great Britain

*This book is dedicated to the loving memory of
Dr. Susan Cooper, who taught me all I need to know
about life, love, motherhood, and new ways of
building families. Her life was a blessing.*
EG

I dedicate this book to my children, Benjamin and Elena.
ES

CONTENTS

ACKNOWLEDGEMENTS

We acknowledge the contributions of the many mothers and fathers through egg donation who have shared their personal stories with us and the professionals who have shared their experience and wisdom and are quoted informally throughout this book. The following people gave generously of their time and expertise: Judy Calica, MSW; Ruth Claiborne, JD; Susan L. Crockin, JD; Joann Paley Galst, PhD; Elaine Gordon, PhD; Carol Fulwiler Jones, MA; Wendy Kramer; Sharon LaMothe; Carol Lesser, NP; Joe B. Massey, MD; Patricia Mendell, LCSW; Olivia Montuschi; Kris Probasco, MSW; Christine Reynolds; Judy Shankman, RN; Ruth Shidlo, PhD; Sanford Benardo, Esq and Jean Kollantai of CLIMB; Carole Lieber Wilkins, MFT; Robin Newman; Ellie Goldman, LICSW; Susan Levin, LICSW; Adele Kauffman, PhD; and Carole Lieber Wilkins, MA. A special thanks goes to Diane Allen of the Infertility Network in Canada, whose tireless work has kept us up to date on matters relating to egg donation worldwide.

I (Ellen) give a special thanks to my husband, Dan Manning, without whose patience, support and computer literacy this book would not exist. I am also grateful to my grandson, Ryan Levesque, who has taught me that the gift of parenthood is a gift that keeps on giving. And, as the dedication of this book reflects, I am ever grateful to my beloved friend and co-author Susan Cooper who died nearly ten years ago but whose wise perspective on family building (and everything else) remains ever with me.

I (Evelina) want to thank my family—Dan, Ben and Ellie—who supported me throughout this process by giving me the time and flexibility to write.

– 1 –

Some Introductions

Most of us grow up expecting that we can and eventually will become parents. We know how it is done—you find a partner you love, make love, get pregnant and nine months later you have a baby. Few people give any thought, initially, to the possibility that their own experience of family building may not be quite that simple. But things happen. Life intervenes. And, if you are reading this book, you have already come to understand that becoming a parent will not be as simple and straightforward as you once thought it would be.

You are not alone in finding that your journey to parenthood—and subsequently, your parenting experience—is different from what you expected it to be. We are keenly aware of how disappointed you may be feeling as you read this. You had hopes, dreams, and expectations and now it seems that they are being dismantled or even shattered. We hope that in the course of reading this book, you will come to a different perspective: that your experience is different but it is not "less than" or "second best." We have known countless women and men struggle as they decide to pursue a second choice path to parenthood, only to land in what they feel is the best place imaginable. This includes many mothers through egg donation who say, once their baby arrives, "I wouldn't have done it any other way. I couldn't love any other baby as much." Several have turned to the words of philosopher Joseph Campbell to capture their experience, "You must give up the life you planned in order to have the life that is waiting for you."

Introducing us—Ellen and Evelina

Before we introduce you to other people whose personal and/or professional lives have been touched by egg donation, we want to introduce ourselves and to say something about how we came to write this book together...

Ellen is a clinical social worker and writer who has been helping people build families for over 30 years. She has a private practice in Newton, Massachusetts, where she focuses on adoption, pregnancy loss, donor conception, surrogacy and parenting after infertility. She is the author of two books, *The Long Awaited Stork: A Guide to Parenting after Infertility* and *Experiencing Infertility: Stories to Inform and Inspire*, and the co-author, with Dr. Susan Cooper, of *Choosing Assisted Reproduction: Social, Emotional and Ethical Considerations*. In addition to her clinical practice and professional writing, Ellen is an essayist and freelance writer.

Evelina is a public health researcher and educator with over 20 years' experience working in the field of reproductive and women's health. She completed her doctorate in the Department of Sociology at Georgia State University in Atlanta, Georgia, as well as a master's degree in public health from the Johns Hopkins University, Baltimore, Maryland. Her research interests include issues related to gender and sexuality, as well as the long-term impacts of infertility. She is the co-author of several other books, including *Living with PCOS—Polycystic Ovary Syndrome*, *Budgeting for Infertility: How to Bring Home a Baby Without Breaking the Bank*, and *Before Your Time: Living Well with Early Menopause*. She has also written several articles specifically addressing family building and infertility.

We are writing this book together and will most often speak as "we." That is not to say that we agree on everything, but, for the most part, we have tried to present material from a shared perspective. However, since we come from different professional backgrounds—clinical social work and public health—there are times when we do bring different perspectives. At those times, when we feel we must say "I" and not "we," we follow the "I" with the speaker's first name (Ellen or Evelina).

The purpose of this book

Not long ago it was unimaginable—the idea that eggs could be transferred from one woman to another. Today it is common. Throughout the world thousands of women have become—and are becoming—mothers through egg donation. Perhaps one day you will be among them.

Egg donation is one of several paths to parenthood that require the use of a third party's reproductive capabilities. These collaborative reproductions include using donated sperm, using donated eggs, surrogacy, using a gestational carrier and embryo placement. For some time these options have been lumped together in both consumer and professional thinking as extensions of medical treatment. In this book we are endorsing a change in perspective. While it is true that medical techniques—insemination, in vitro fertilization (IVF) or perhaps other assisted reproductive technologies (ARTs)—are required for conception in collaborative reproduction, conception is far from the end of the journey when families are built by collaborative reproductive options. We believe that it is vital that families making these choices not consider them extensions of treatment, but that they understand that, in choosing a collaborative reproductive option, they are embarking on a psychosocial and emotional journey with lifelong consequences for all involved—would-be parents, third-party participants and, most of all, the children brought into the world as a result of collaborative reproduction. We believe that collaborative reproduction should be thought of as a psychosocial as well as a medical issue.

Unlike many books about the infertility experience, this is not a book centered on medicine and treatment. While we will offer limited medical information that would-be parents need to have to make informed decisions, our basic focus in *Having Your Baby Through Egg Donation* is on the psychosocial ramifications of having and parenting a baby using the eggs of a donor. While the book presents many facts, it does not claim to be objective. Our book contains the strong, experientially informed opinions of its authors.

We have written this book as a guide to your journey toward making decisions about whether or not to use donated eggs. Whatever brings you to consider egg donation, we assume that the experience has not been easy. We hope that this book will offer you comfort, guidance, information and support as you make your way. We hope, also, that it will remind you that you are not alone. Others have traveled this path before you, and many women and men traverse it now.

Here, in the introduction, we introduce you to one family—the Gordons. We have selected them for our introduction because their story and their perspective cover the central themes in this book. As with all the families who have shared their stories with us, we have changed their names, geographical location and occupations in order to respect their privacy. We have not changed key facts central to their story.

Meet Carla, Rob, Rebecca, Jennifer, Jake and Matt

A visitor arriving at Carla and Rob Gordon's home has an immediate reaction: KIDS! The Gordons' spacious front porch is filled with bikes, sporting equipment, a double stroller. A glance to the back yard reveals a swing set and a trampoline. *This is a busy family*, one thinks. *This is a home filled with kids.*

And indeed it is, but it was not always this way. Fifteen years ago, when Carla and Rob bought an old colonial farmhouse in what was then a quiet, rural town about 65 miles north of Boston, they were looking forward to having a child. Then another. They were 26 years old, recently married, newly minted master's-trained teachers who chose to buy in "Rutherford" (we are changing all names to protect privacy) because it was affordable, had good schools and seemed to be an all-round fine place to raise a family. First came love, then came marriage, then came the house and now for the baby carriage.

Like many couples who come upon infertility unexpectedly, Carla and Rob were initially baffled when Carla did not conceive. After all, they were young, led very healthy lives, had no family history of infertility and had been dutifully using birth control since first they met. *Who us?* they thought. *Not us. We were made to have babies.*

And they certainly were, but not yet. When they had been trying to for a year, Carla sought medical attention, assuming that the problem was hers. Fortunately, her physician did not make the same mistake and told her that before he did any testing on her, he wanted Rob to do a semen analysis. "After all," Carla's physician said, "it is the man about half the time."

And indeed it was, but not entirely. Rob was tested and the couple was told that he had a very low sperm count—so low, in fact, that it was "fruitless" for the couple to try to conceive with Rob's sperm. The Gordons were stunned and upset that anyone could dismiss Rob's paternity so cavalierly and usher them on to donor sperm "as if it were nothing."

In fact, thinking about donor sperm was hardly nothing! Carla and Rob remember spending several months thinking about donor insemination (DI), all the while "hoping the doctor was wrong and that we'd get pregnant on our own." But that didn't happen, Carla and Rob spent a good deal of time talking about what it would mean to have a child that was genetically connected to Carla but not to Rob, especially since Carla would carry the child for nine months. After a time the Gordons realized that they were beginning to feel receptive to the idea of using donor sperm. It was time to pick a donor.

When they made the decision to use donor sperm, Carla and Rob felt a sense of relief. "We'd done all the hard work—or so we thought." The couple felt certain that deciding on donor sperm was the difficult part and that picking a donor would be an easier task. The process of decision making had brought them closer together, and both approached donor selection with optimism. "We'd have some fun with it. We'd look at profiles closely. We'd find someone we really wanted to have as a part of our family."

The Gordons' sense of fun and optimism carried them only so far and lasted only so long. The couple, who had expected to conceive easily on their own, now anticipated conceiving immediately with the first donor they selected. Neither could ever have anticipated trying with three donors and going through a series of fertility treatments all the way up to IVF.

"Eventually, we did conceive, and by that time it practically didn't matter that it was with donor sperm," says Rob. He remembers just wanting a baby and not caring so much how the baby came. But, for Carla, it was different. She recalls being pregnant with the couple's first daughter, Rebecca, and worrying that Rob wouldn't love this baby.

When Rebecca was born and Rob was not as involved and attentive as Carla was, she worried that her fears had come to pass. It was not until one day—a week or two into motherhood—that she burst into tears and said, "I'm so sad that you don't love her." What a relief it was for Carla when Rob looked at her, baffled and confused, and said, "Of course I do. Of course I do."

And, of course, he did. Rob and Rebecca were close from the start and remain so, even as Rebecca, now 11, heads towards adolescence. For Carla, watching her husband and their firstborn share such a strong bond has been a source of great joy and relief. Her pleasure has increased all the more since the couple's second daughter, Jennifer, came along. Jennifer was not conceived with donor sperm: Rob is her biological father.

So how did that happen, you ask? Thrilled with Rebecca, Carla and Rob returned to the fertility clinic that had "given us our daughter" and requested "the same again." They wanted the same donor, the same treatment and hoped for the same outcome. To their surprise, the physician responded to their request with a very different recommendation: "I know that we told you something different a few years ago, but with the use of ICSI—intracytoplasmic sperm injection, where a single sperm is injected into the egg for fertilization—we believe that you can probably conceive with Rob's sperm."

This news startled Rob and Carla as much as the original bleak pronouncement had a few years earlier. They were, however, happy to take the doctor up on his offer to try IVF with Rob's sperm. Fortunate to live in Massachusetts, which has enjoyed an insurance mandate since 1985, the Gordons did not have to worry about the cost of treatment. Insurance would cover IVF and ICSI, and if treatment didn't work, there was nothing ventured, nothing lost financially. They would simply turn to DI again. DI had blessed them with a wonderful first child, and Rob and Carla were certain that it would work again.

This time around it wasn't going to be quite so difficult. The first IVF cycle didn't bring a pregnancy, but it did bring nice evidence of fertilization. The same thing was true the second time around. "We were a little discouraged, but our experience trying to get pregnant a few years earlier had taught us that patience and fortitude pay off."

And indeed they did. Carla was pregnant on the third IVF-ICSI cycle, and she gave birth to Jennifer nine months later.

"Was it amazing for you to be the biological father to your child?" we asked Rob.

"No," he replied. "What was amazing was to see her born at home. Rebecca was there too and she was very much a part of things."

A home birth is hardly something that most infertile couples aspire to. "Give me the lights, the instruments, the cast of thousands and all the machines," many veterans of infertility declare. Many—but not Carla Gordon. For Carla, who hates to take so much as an aspirin, the whole high-tech trip through infertility had been difficult—"something I had to cope with because I wanted a baby so much." Now, with a healthy, uneventful pregnancy, she was determined to have as natural an experience as she could—a home birth followed by a long period of nursing.

When Jennifer was four years old, baby fever struck again. Although Carla and Rob had initially anticipated having two children and had felt prepared to "bargain for one" before Rebecca was born, their struggles with infertility had altered their sense of family. "We had come to appreciate what an incredible miracle every child is and we wanted more. The only problem was that I had just about aged out of the picture."

Carla, 26 when it all began, was 40 when she and Rob returned to the fertility center for yet another try. "By this time they had declared that Rob was just fine, but I could see that the doctor was worried about my eggs. He did an FSH and a clomiphene citrate challenge test and came back with news that was remarkably similar to the news we had gotten about Rob nearly 14 years earlier. "You are wasting time to try on your own. You should use donor eggs."

"Donor eggs? When I heard the words, I wasn't the least bit upset—I was ecstatic. The recommendation sent my heart soaring. After all, we'd long ago made peace with the idea of having a child through donor gametes. That work had been done, and we had a wonderful child to show for it. What sent my heart soaring was the news that egg donors were now available. When we had gone through donor sperm, I remembered hearing that women were on waiting lists for years for donor eggs."

"'No, it's become easy to locate a donor,' our doctor told us. He put us in touch with a lawyer who specializes in finding donors and helps match them with recipients. We made an appointment and eagerly piled the girls into the car for what would be the newest Gordon family project," Carla continues. "The lawyer was lovely but when he saw the children, he seemed a little surprised and confused. He pointed to them and asked how we could look at donor profiles when our children were with us. 'Oh, they came to help us,' I explained. Then he looked really surprised."

Indeed, Rebecca and Jennifer were there to help their parents select a donor. Needless to say, the real choice would be the parents' decision, but Rebecca and Jennifer, who have both known about their own origins for as long as they can remember, wanted to be part of things. For them, it is entirely natural for families to be created in all sorts of ways and for parents to talk openly and honestly with their children about assisted reproduction and gamete donation.

Carla and Rob found a donor they liked. They were pleased to find that egg donation—at least with their lawyer—was more open than sperm donation had been for them. They were able to talk with their donor and to exchange letters and pictures in a non-identifying way. The process was set in motion, and, to Carla and Rob's surprise, Carla was pregnant on the first cycle. But there was to be a bigger surprise up ahead.

When Carla and Rob learned that she was carrying twins, they were stunned. Having spent over a decade in reproductive medicine, they were well aware that twins were always a possibility, but, as Rob put it, "We weren't surprised, we were shocked."

Last year Carla gave birth to baby boys, Jake and Matt. When asked how this—her donor egg pregnancy—felt different to the others, Carla comments first on the fact that it was twins, then on the fact that she felt like an "old mother"—and only then on the fact that the twins came from a donor.

"I felt that if I couldn't give them my genes, I could grow them as best I could. I did everything I could to eat well, rest well, take care of myself and to carry them as long as I could." Carla goes on to add that she carried the twins until 39 weeks and gave birth to them vaginally. And if that is not remarkable enough, the twins weighed 8 pounds 3 ounces and 6 pounds 13 ounces at birth!

And so that is how the Gordons' front porch came to exclaim "Kids!" It doesn't announce "Donor sperm" or "Donor egg" or "IVF" or "ICSI." The bikes and sporting equipment and the double stroller, like life inside the home, say that this is what it is—a normal, natural, content and thriving family.

"But what do the kids think?" you might be wondering. "How do the children cope with information about donor insemination or egg donation? And how could the parents have been brave enough to tell them? I wouldn't be that brave," you fear.

Carla and Rob do not see themselves as brave, nor do they see their children as suffering, in any way, from knowing how their family came to be. Rather, the Gordons feel that the topic is one to be handled honestly and openly with their children. Moreover, they are happy to tell all of their children how much they wanted them, how hard they worked to have them, how grateful they are to the donors who helped them and, above all, how thrilled they are to be their parents. It is a joyous story, and one that is revisited in different ways, at different times.

As open as the Gordons have been at home, both are clear that the story of how their family came to be is a private matter. Beyond their minister, their reproductive endocrinologist, their obstetrician and Rob's mother, who learned because Rebecca told her, almost no one knows what Rob and Carla did to create their family. "We feel it is the children's private information and it is theirs to share, as they wish, when they wish." Thus far, Rebecca, the only Gordon child really old enough to talk about donor conception with others, has chosen to keep her story private.

When asked if they have any regrets, the Gordons smile and say, "No, only gratitude." But then Carla pauses for a moment and speaks a truth about the legacy of infertility. "I have a terrific family. I'm having a blast. I couldn't be happier, but I'll admit, I still wonder what it would be like to just find myself pregnant. I know it is a pipe dream at this point, as my eggs are old and I know that our lives are full with children, but how amazing, how wonderful it would be to just one day wake up and find myself pregnant." With this Carla pauses for a moment and then jumps up: one of the twins is crying and it is time to pick up Jennifer from school.

We thank the Gordons for introducing several of the themes that run through this book. As Carla Gordon put it, "Our family spans the history of modern infertility treatment."

Reproductive medicine is a changing field

Indeed, reproductive medicine is a changing field. Rob Gordon, the biological father of three children, was once told he would never father a child. Carla Gordon, in her mid-20s when she first attempted pregnancy, never anticipated she would be turning to an egg donor as she neared 40. We cannot begin to fathom the changes that will occur between now and the time the Gordon children are ready to start families of their own.

Our central themes

While every family's decision to have their baby through egg donation is uniquely their own, we have found there are several overarching themes that many experience similarly.

People make decisions based on their changing reality

Egg donation is often an unexpected journey. Although there are those among you who have anticipated egg donation for many years, the majority of women who conceive through donated eggs never expected to travel this path.

People come to egg donation after loss. You learn you were born without ovaries; you learn your eggs are "old" (even if *you* are not); you lose your ovarian function because of chemotherapy. Things happen. Your reality changes, and, as it does, you come to see your options through a different lens.

Throughout this book we will remind you repeatedly to "never say never."

Again, the Gordons' story is illustrative. When I (Ellen) first met Carla and Rob, they had just learned of Rob's infertility. As a couple, they were first grappling with questions of donor sperm. If someone had told them then that, even with donor sperm, they would have to try IVF three times, they would have exclaimed, "Never!" Surely, if someone had told them that Rob's sperm would be capable of fertilizing an egg, they would have exclaimed "Never!" in total bafflement. And, no doubt, the information that their third and fourth children would be conceived through egg donation would have startled them. You get the picture: their reality changed and, with it, their perspective.

You are the architects of your family story and the proud owners of that story

If you choose egg donation, you have the opportunity to formulate your family story. Unlike adoptive parents, who build on a story that is already underway, parents via egg donation make decisions, from the start, that design the story. Throughout this book we will encourage you to look to the future and, in particular, to your hoped-for child's feelings, as you make the decisions that will begin your child's story.

Making decisions you feel good about should pay off in many ways. In addition to providing you with confidence as you begin conversations with your child, you should also feel comfortable talking—or not talking—with others. As owners of your family story, it is for you to decide when you want to talk about donor conception and when you do not.

When we both first began working in egg donation in the mid-1990s, there was a climate of secrecy. Sadly, the very people who worked so hard to build their families were slinking around as though they had a shameful secret. Thanks, in large measure, to the outspoken voices of adopted children and those through sperm donation, attitudes are changing. We now live in a time in which parents through egg donation feel a greater sense of confidence and legitimacy.

Why are open conversations with children so important? We have long believed that without openness, there is the risk that egg donation will feel shameful. We worried that parents who did not speak openly with their children would prompt their children to feel that their birth was "second best," that their parents felt they had "something to hide," that there was a "missing piece" in their lives. Recently, researchers Bohanek, Marin, Fivush, and Duke at Emory University have offered even more compelling reasons for talking openly with children. They developed a 20 question, "Do you know?" scale and found that children who know the most about their family history, score highest in self-confidence. The authors write, "We experience many important and emotional events with our families, and reminiscing about these shared experiences who we are both within the family and as individuals" (2006). Included in the "Do you know" questions are questions about how their parents' dealt with adversity such as illness or accidents. Tellingly, there is the question, "Do you know the story of your birth?"

Being open and honest does not mean, however, that parents through egg donation should self-consciously announce to everyone, "I had my child through egg donation," or, worse, refer to their baby as "my egg donor baby." Rather, we recommend that people talk about egg donation on a "reason to tell" or "reason to talk" basis. We encourage parents to tell others how their child was conceived *if* there is a reason to tell them. We remind you that you are not only creating your family story, but you are also determining how and when that story will be told and to whom.

Acting in the best interests of children

Reproductive medicine exists to create children for people who want to parent them. These would-be parents are the clients of reproductive medicine centers and, in many instances, of gamete donation programs. Nonetheless, the primary concern should not be to please would-be parents nor the women who offer to help them. Rather, attention should always be paid—first and foremost—to the well-being of children. In the case of egg donation, we are often talking about unborn children.

Throughout this book we pay close attention to the best interests of children. Adults, whether they are recipient couples or egg donors, should be capable of making informed decisions for themselves. But who speaks for the children? Their rights must be attended to and protected. Among these rights we include the right to know the truth about their origins, the right to information about their genetic ancestry, the right to privacy, the right of access to one's genetic relatives and the right to parents who are of childrearing age.

This last right is increasingly difficult to define. When we raised this question in the first edition of this book, we received criticism from some older parents who felt we were biased. We took this criticism seriously and examined it, trying to distinguish between what may be personal bias and what may truly be in the best interests—or not—of children. Our conversations, between ourselves and with others, have led to a more flexible approach in this book, recognizing that there are many benefits to older parenting.

People feel differently about genetics and gestation

Women who donate eggs, whether to family members, friends or strangers, are able to do so because they do not see an egg as "their child." When asked what the egg means to them, they will often liken it to blood—a valuable and useful part of their bodies that they can give to someone else because they do not need it.

Not everyone feels this way. There are many women who say they "could never give away my genetic material." Often these same women can say with confidence, "I'd be happy to carry someone else's baby for them, but I could never give them my eggs."

Our point is that people feel very differently about genetics and gestational ties. For some, all that really matters are the genetic ties—these are the links to generations past and future. To others, it is the act of pregnancy—of gestating a child and giving birth—that really matters.

It is important, as you read this book, for you to think about how you feel about genes and gestation. There is no right or wrong, better or worse. We are simply acknowledging the natural differences among people. You need to understand where you are on the genes/gestation spectrum *and* where your partner is. Only then can you face decisions about egg donation clearly and honestly. If genetic ties are crucial to you, you may be most comfortable with an intrafamily donation if one is available to you. Or you may decide to pursue adoption, feeling "it is only fair that if one of us cannot have a genetic tie to our child, neither of us can."

The Gordon family represents a spectrum of genetic and gestational bonds. Carla has gestational ties to all four of her children but genetic ties to two. Rob, who was prepared to parent without any genetic ties to his children, ended up with genetic links to three of his four children. The parents and the children are aware of the differences that exist in the family, but, as Carla explains it, these differences are simply there. For example, she feels a touch of pleasure when Rebecca comments on how much she and Jake—who share no genetic link—look alike.

Carrying and delivering a baby forges strong bonds

Having just acknowledged that genes are of paramount importance to some people and of relatively less importance to others, we turn to the significance of pregnancy. Even those who would choose a genetic connection over a gestational one, if they could make that choice, often find that carrying a child for nine months—or sharing a pregnancy with one's partner for nine months—forges powerful bonds. Carla Gordon, who shared a genetic connection with her first two children, spoke to this bond when she so proudly affirmed, "I grew their hearts, I grew their brains, and I fed them for nine months and grew them with all the love I could possibly give."

Epigenetics and microchimerism are two fairly recent concepts that fortify the significance of gestational bonds. Epigenetics is the study of heritable changes in gene expression or cellular phenotype caused by mechanisms other than changes in the underlying DNA sequence. Microchimerism is the presence of a small number of cells that originate in one individual and cross the placenta into another. Women pregnant through egg donation are often comforted to know that their cells will live on in their child for years to come.

Couples can strengthen their relationships as they journey through infertility and gamete donation

"Whatever doesn't break us will make us stronger." This certainly applies to infertility, which is, for most couples, a devastating life crisis. Although some relationships may crumble under the stress of infertility, many are strengthened. Surely the process of exploring and possibly attempting an egg donor pregnancy has the potential to strengthen a relationship. The process forces people to take a serious look at why they want to be parents together, how they will share a parenthood that is not genetically equal, how they will respect the importance of privacy while avoiding the hazards of secrecy.

Pregnancy and parenthood through egg donation are legitimate and authentic

If you choose egg donation, you should do so believing that you have a right to this decision and to the child or children it brings into your life. Sadly, we meet women who work so hard to conceive through egg donation but react to a positive pregnancy test by feeling "fake." Although this feeling seems to diminish as a pregnancy unfolds, some feelings of being not-quite-a-real-parent linger, sometimes even after a child is born. We remind you again of Carla Gordon's affirming words: "I grew their hearts, I grew their brains." If you make this choice and if it works, *you* will grow your baby. More important still, *you* will raise this child. You'll be the tooth fairy and the carpool pick-up and the one who lies awake at night when your newly minted driver is out on the road. If that isn't real parenthood, we don't know what is!

Look ahead, not behind

"We shouldn't have waited so long," "I shouldn't have focused so much on my career." "My husband and I should have met earlier," "We shouldn't have waited until we had a house…" And on it goes. Regrets? All too often, they are heavy and unnecessary burdens. We remind you that none of us make decisions planning to one day regret them. If you move forward with egg donation, try to cast off the demons of regret and focus instead on the path that lies ahead.

Now that we've trashed regret, we want to put in a bit of a good word for it—or at least for "anticipatory regret." By this we refer to making decisions with an eye towards what one might later regret. The question of anticipatory regret arises in egg donation when it comes to donor selection, costs, anonymity. As you confront important decisions regarding egg donation, pause along the way and think about how you—or your future child— may feel about those decisions in the future.

The meaning of donor conception changes over time

When they first think about having a baby through egg donation, many people struggle with the concept. Women fear they will not feel like "real" mothers. This is a concern that remains with many, even well into parenthood. However, as time passes, as diapers are changed, these concerns are likely to fade and others arise. Dr. Maggie Kirkman, an Australian psychologist and researcher who has interviewed many women who are mothers through egg donation, confirms: "One of the most notable findings in my research is the way in which the meaning of donor assisted conception, including egg donation, changes over time and according to what else is happening in the family's life" (Kirkman 2003a). As she picks up toys scattered about, rushes to drive carpool and hurries to get to soccer practice, Carla Gordon will certainly agree that her focus has changed!

The people you meet along the way will shape your journey

As you consider egg donation, you will be talking with physicians, nurses, mental health counselors, parents through egg donation and, possibly, egg donors. The things people say to you and the approaches they take to this decision will influence your decision making. You will also be influenced by the comments— knowing and unknowing—of friends, family and acquaintances. Ultimately, you will be making your own decision, but it would be foolish for us to suggest that that decision is made in a vacuum.

Finances and geography will influence your decisions

As if infertility wasn't enough, people considering egg donation often face geographical and financial challenges. Depending upon the laws in the state or country where you live, egg donation may be more or less available to you. If you live in Italy, you will have to travel internationally to pursue this option. Should you seek anonymous donation and live in the UK, you might need to travel to Spain, the Czech Republic or another country that still permits anonymous donors. If you live in the US, in a state that mandates health insurance coverage for egg donation, the process may be comfortably within your reach.

The blessing and curse of the "meant to be"

"Oh, it was meant to be," well-intentioned people declare upon hearing a couple has had a miscarriage. Or you may say to yourselves, "Maybe we were not meant to be parents." Both are examples of what we call "the curse of the meant to be." How cruel is it to declare that someone who deeply desires a child is not "meant to be" a parent?

On the other hand, there is a blessing of the "meant to be." The blessing comes when things unfold in an unexpected way and the outcome, although not the one originally intended, is a good one. You have twins through donor eggs. They are wonderful. It was meant to be. You adopt a little girl from China. She captivates you and you are certain it was meant to be.

The Chinese believe that there is a tiny, not quite visible, red thread that connects people who belong together. The blessing of the "meant to be" and a belief in "the red thread" offer comfort.

Some other things you should know about this book

Our readers

Although we would be delighted to hear that this book was helpful to a range of readers, we have written it with certain populations in mind. We assume that most of our readers will be women who have learned, for various reasons, that they are unable to become pregnant using their own eggs. We hope that their husbands or partners will also read this book and, perhaps, that they will share it will family members, especially if the family is involved in intrafamily donation.

We are both in the US (although in different cities and regions) and, hence, much of our reference point is the US. However, we have spoken with people around the world for this book and have included their voices and perspectives within it.

Our language

We are aware that some people object to the use of the word *donor* when a woman receives payment, even if it seems clear that the payment is for her time and effort. Some would advise us to say *provider* rather than *donor*. Although we feel that there are instances in which *provider* is the more appropriate term, we like to believe that the majority of women who give their eggs to someone else do see it as a gift. The word *donor* appears to honor that gift more than does the word *provider*.

On the other hand, we will not use the word *disclosure*. This word is often used in reference to truth telling with children. To us, the word *disclosure* implies a secret. Since we see no secret, we will simply say—again and again—that we feel parents need to be truthful with their children.

Perhaps the biggest semantic challenge we faced in writing this book was figuring out how to refer to those egg donors who are neither family members nor friends. They have often been called *anonymous donors*, but since we have reservations about them remaining anonymous to their recipients and to the offspring, this word did not seem an apt description. Nor did we want to call them *paid donors*, since the fees they receive are considered compensation for time and effort, not payment for eggs. Similarly, *commercial donors* did not seem right. Since all donors enter into contracts, the term *contractual donors* didn't work, either. Finally, we decided that the clearest term to distinguish between those donors who were friends or family members of their recipients beforehand and those who did not know their recipients beforehand was to refer to the way in which they were located and matched with a recipient—by being recruited by a medical practice or agency program. We will refer to them as *program-recruited donors*.

Often you will hear the technical words *oocytes, ova* and *ovum* referring to human eggs. While these are the correct words medically, we have chosen to use the colloquial *egg* in this edition and to always refer to the process as *egg donation*.

We refer to the process by which an embryo that originates in one family is transferred to another as *embryo placement*, as opposed to *embryo donation* or *embryo adoption*.

Finally, rather than using the cumbersome "he or she" and "his or her," we have, in most cases, referred to the child born through egg donation as "he." This has also helped to clarify meaning when we refer, in the same sentence, to the mother or egg donor as "she."

This book is meant to be both challenging and supportive. We hope you will enjoy it and find it helpful.

– 2 –
An Overview of
Egg Donation

Egg donation is changing the way we think about family building. Now that gestational and genetic motherhood can be separated, young women born without ovaries can carry, deliver and parent children conceived with another woman's eggs. Women who survive cancer at the expense of their fertility are able to experience pregnancy and the joy of bringing new life into the world. Women can extend their fertility beyond their biological clocks. New families are being formed, together with new definitions of kinship.

Egg donation is still evolving, and, should you choose this path, you will be part of its early history. In this chapter we attempt to provide you with a context in which to view egg donation, past, present and future. From there we will move on to the "departure lounge of egg donation" so that you can meet your fellow travelers.

Historical perspective

So how did it all begin? There are published records from as early as the late 1800s of experiments conducted on women who lost their ovaries at a young age. However, it was not until the arrival of in vitro fertilization (IVF) in 1978 that physicians had a means for enabling a woman to become pregnant with another woman's eggs. The first child conceived through egg donation was born in Australia in 1983.

In its early years egg donation, though possible, was not readily available. The first donors were either sisters or cousins of their recipients or they were infertile women who were undergoing IVF. Since cryopreservation of embryos was not available to all, some of these women had extra eggs for which they had only two options: discard or donate to other infertile women. Another group of early egg donors were women seeking tubal ligation who were invited to donate their eggs in exchange for the cost of their procedure. Either way, donated eggs were relatively few and far between and, for the most part, came from women whose donation was based more on practicality or expediency than on an affirmative decision to help an infertile couple. The scarcity of eggs made the experience challenging for would-be recipients who had little way of knowing if and when donated eggs would become available to them. One mother of a now 23-year-old through egg donation recalls taking medications over an extended period of time to ensure her uterus was ready for implantation should a donated egg come along. She was literally "on call" for news that an egg was available. When the call came, there was no asking about who the donor was or what her genetic history revealed. The recipient was instructed to go immediately to the fertility clinic where she underwent a full laparatomy (a surgical incision in the abdominal area) and a gamete intrafallopian transfer (GIFT procedure) in which the donor's eggs were mixed with the recipient's husband's sperm and placed in her tubes.

Much has changed. Not only has IVF fully replaced GIFT as a vehicle for egg donation, but, beginning in the late 1980s, women were actively recruited for voluntary egg donation. This began in medical clinics, some of whom continue to recruit donors. However, in the United States, independent egg donor agencies rapidly replaced medical programs as the main source of donated eggs. By the late 1990s it was common to see advertisements like the following in college newspapers:

Make a dream come true. Help a childless couple become parents. If you are under 34, healthy, a non-smoker, please consider donating some of your eggs. You will be compensated for your time and effort.

The arrival of these programs transformed egg donation from something extremely difficult to arrange to something that, with financial/health insurance resources and access to medical treatment, can be launched with a few visits to internet websites. One need simply type in "egg donation" to be connected to agencies with names ranging from Precious Wonders to Tiny Treasures to An Angel's Gift to Peas in a Pod and Our Fairy Godmother. At the time of writing, there are nearly 100 egg donor agencies listed on the website of the American Society for Reproductive Medicine (ASRM). Most have tantalizing websites that offer hope to infertile couples, many of whose journey to parenthood has so far been filled with only disappointment and loss. They also offer the promise of financial and emotional reward to young women who are invited to undergo ovarian stimulation and egg retrieval.

Just as there have been changes in the availability and accessibility of donors, so also have there been shifts in the way people think about egg donation. In the early years there was a real sense that the science was advancing far more rapidly than our understanding of what it means for a person to be physically born to three people. Instead of taking note of what a seismic shift this marked in human reproduction, physicians presented egg donation as a treatment for female infertility. In so doing, they missed the opportunity to examine, make sense of and ultimately celebrate what egg donation means for identity formation and our understanding of kinship. Sadly, egg donation was pushed into the shadows, spoken of in hushed tones and burdened by secrecy.

The experiences of parents through egg donation, their children and their donors changed significantly with the arrival of the Donor Sibling Registry (DSR) in 2000. This US-based worldwide registry was founded in 2000 by Wendy Kramer and her son, Ryan, who was conceived through sperm donation. The registry helps people connect with donor relations. In the 13 years since its founding, the DSR has helped connect more than 9200 individuals with their donor relations. Wendy Kramer reports there are on average two new matches every day. For egg donation families, this has meant that parents have connected with donors, donors with offspring and, as the name of the DSR suggests, offspring with other offspring. As word of the DSR has grown, and, with it, people's appreciation of the significance of genetic connections, families have been turning to the DSR in new ways. Currently, there are several egg donor agencies in the US that include the DSR in their donor-recipient contracts, making it possible for people who want anonymity (or at least to start out with no identifying information) to remain in touch and share photos and updated medical and social information. The DSR's global presence is growing steadily, with membership coming from around the world and in large numbers from Canada, Australia, Spain, Romania and Israel.

Where are we today?

Looking at egg donation today, we see a very different picture from what we saw even as recently as the original (2005) edition of *Having Your Baby Through Egg Donation*. In addition to the changes noted above, we see changes in the way egg donation (ED) parents feel about their path to parenthood. The secrecy that prevailed in the past has diminished significantly. True, there are some ED parents who still feel they have something to be secretive about, but increasing numbers are treating their child's story as an open but private matter. They don't go around saying "my egg donor baby," but acknowledge donor conception when there is a reason to do so. In talking about it in a natural and appropriate way, most find that others are fully accepting of and comfortable with egg donation. Accompanying this more open approach to egg donation in general has been increased comfort with the donors. As one mother through egg donation put it:

> When I first heard about egg donation, I did not want to meet my donor because I thought that I would see her face in my child and it would upset me. Now I feel the opposite. I have twins and one looks just like the donor. I love it because it is a constant reminder of the remarkable woman who helped make us a family.

With increased comfort and familiarity with egg donation has come increased use of this option. Or perhaps it is the reverse: as more people have become parents through egg donation, more of them have become comfortable speaking openly about it. Either way, the use of egg donation is on the rise. In 2010, the Society for Assisted Reproductive Technology (SART) reported there were 9321 transfers using donated eggs. Over 55 percent of these resulted in live births. This is the official SART number. Wendy Kramer of the DSR found, in surveying parents through egg donation, that 42 percent were never asked to inform their clinic whether they had a live birth. Some did so voluntarily and others did not. If we add in the pregnancies that resulted from cryopreserved embryo transfers, there were more than 8000 births in the US in 2010 alone from donated eggs.

A current trend in the United States is the promotion of "egg banks." Until recently, it was difficult to freeze human eggs, and few documented pregnancies resulted from eggs that had been frozen. The development of vitrification, an effective means of freezing and thawing eggs, has made it possible for women to freeze eggs for future use. As vitirication has been developed and improved, with reports of pregnancy rates between 54 percent and 63 percent per transfer, egg banks have become a source of donated eggs. We are hearing of more and more reproductive medicine centers partnering with egg banks and offering patients egg donation at one-third the cost and a much faster process.

Challenges remain—ethical, legal and regulatory concerns

Reproductive technology and egg donation practice are moving at such a rapid pace today that many important social, ethical and legal considerations are lagging behind significantly. Many of us, including leaders in the field of reproductive technology, are unsure what the next steps should be.

Although egg donation has enjoyed widespread acceptance and relatively little scrutiny in the United States, this is not the case throughout the world. In Italy, for instance, a law was passed in 2004 to ban egg donation completely, banning also the use of donor sperm and helping women past childbearing age becoming pregnant via ARTs. The road to this law started in 1994 when Italy made headlines because Dr. Severino Antinori used donor eggs to allow 63-year-old Rosana Della Cortes to become pregnant. Robin Marantz Henig states:

> We are learning the wrong lessons from our earlier misadventures. Things got a little out of hand, yes, but that is because governments around the world adopted a hands-off policy towards the whole affair. It was too complicated to reach consensus about what steps were too intrusive, about when human life begins, about what risks were worth taking for the sake of having one's own biological child. So governments turned their backs on reproductive technology and allowed the field to be taken over by cowboys. (Henig 2004)

Still unable to come to a consensus about exactly what should and should not be accepted with regard to egg donation, countries such as Italy, Austria, Norway, Sweden and Switzerland have also nearly eliminated egg donation. While such strict laws serve to call everyone's attention to the potential for ethical abuses in egg donation, they also create new social problems. There now exists what has been termed "fertility tourism"—people living in countries that ban egg donation are traveling to other countries to obtain eggs.

Many counties in which IVF and other ARTs are part of national health care plans—such as France, the Netherlands, Spain, the United Kingdom, Canada and Australia—have legislation in place regulating egg donation. These policies especially place restrictions on anonymous donors. The Human Fertilisation and Embryology Authority (HFEA) is a government body in the UK which regulates and inspects all clinics providing IVF and donor conception. Its governing board, which includes people who have had personal experience of donor conception, along with experts in the field of reproductive medicine and bioethics, makes important decisions regarding regulations about the way donor conception is carried out. In January 2003 the UK announced a registry for donor offspring, which was established in 2004 as a pilot project. This voluntary registry enables donor offspring and donors who participated in gamete donation before 1991, when the Human Fertilisation and Embryology Act came into being, to exchange information. Since then more than 18,000 children have been born in the United Kingdom with donated gametes. In 2004 the United Kingdom also announced that, after April 2005, anyone looking to donate eggs or sperm would no longer be given anonymity. Similarly, some Scandinavian countries have always had open sperm donor files, and clinics in New Zealand do not accept anonymous donors.

Another worldwide difference of note is the use of IVF patients as a source of egg donation or egg sharing. This is allowed and even promoted in Canada, Denmark, India, Israel, Spain and the United Kingdom, as well as sometimes in the United States. Many European countries, particularly those that support egg sharing, provide government funding to women attempting anywhere between two and five cycles of IVF. Many feel that this method of engaging egg sharing among government-funded IVF cycles ensures "more bang for the government's buck." On the other hand, New Zealand believes that egg donors are only able to give consent without the pressures of financial incentives; as a result, egg donors are not allowed to be paid in any case.

The *New York Times* has an "Ask the Ethicist" column each Sunday in its magazine section. Evidence of how mainstream egg donation has become came on April 8, 2012, when the column concerned egg donation. Specifically, the writer complains about a "fertility consultant" who took their money and then failed to search for an egg donor with a Hawaiian background. The ethicist chooses to comment more on the intended parents' desires to find a donor of their ethnicity than on the fact that, in the US, anyone can call themselves a fertility consultant or an egg donor agency and charge large sums of money to find egg donors.

It is seems odd to us that even in the "Ask the Ethicist" column, the ethicist does not address some of the fundamental ethical concerns of egg donation: should women be paid? If so, how much? Should anonymous donation be permitted? How should egg donation be regulated and by whom?

It seems that the most controversial issue worldwide involves financial compensation to donors. There are countries, such as Australia and Canada, that prohibit payment to donors and there are others, such as the UK, that limit payments to a compensation for time spent. By contrast, the United States has allowed an industry to develop in which donors commonly receive between $5000 and $10,000 and, all too often, upwards of $15,000. Although the American Society for Reproductive Medicine (ASRM) stipulates that this payment is for time and effort, women are commonly receiving higher payments when they have donated successfully in previous cycles. One would think that, if anything, a second- or third-time donor would spend less time and effort on the cycle, since she is familiar with the process, but, rather than her fee remaining the same or being reduced, it rises with each successful cycle. Similarly, women who are physically beautiful or have high SAT scores may also command higher fees, again suggesting that the payment is not simply for time and effort.

Major ethical issues range from concern for the offspring, some of whom may be forever separated from their genetic relatives, to concerns for the donors, who may be enticed by the payments to do something they may later regret, to concerns for the recipients, some of whom may be entering into parenthood at advanced age with inadequate understanding of the challenges involved for themselves or their children.

Other questions about egg donation involve who should regulate the practice and how it should it be regulated. Some in the United States feel that this country should follow in the footsteps of nations that have implemented governmental regulations and restrictions. Others in the United States prefer to have professional organizations, such as those in the field of reproductive medicine, responsible for making these types of decisions, rather than government agencies. Still others argue that since egg donation is a multidisciplinary field, it, should be thoughtfully guided by a panel of experts in medicine, science, genetics, psychology, sociology, theology and law. They feel that these professionals can work together for a common goal: to maintain excellent quality of care while considering the effects on greater society.

Regardless of who regulates egg donation, the questions around regulation all involve protecting the best interests of all participants. First, the offspring. The appreciation for the lifelong impact of donation on all participants has come largely from a worldwide movement of donor offspring (although all adult donor offspring were conceived through donated sperm, not egg donation, they do not differentiate themselves from anonymous egg donor offspring). Many donor offspring throughout the world have spoken poignantly and powerfully about their experiences.

Christine Whipp wrote an article entitled "Why I need to find my father" in which she writes:

> Luckily through the media and the internet I came into contact with other donor offspring from across the globe... It soon became apparent that we share a commonality in our experiences and have identified many uncomfortable issues with which we must deal as a result of the choices made by our parents. These can include feelings of revulsion at the clinical method by which we were produced; a sense of loss and grief for deliberately severed relationships with unknown biological kinfolk; a fear of accidental incest; anger and frustration at the lack of respect shown for our missing genetic origins and the indescribable emotional burdens which we carry as part of an inherited compromise. (Whipp 2004)

Many donor-conceived adults will freely admit that their sense of identity has been damaged and would concur with Cicero that: "To be ignorant of what occurred before you were born is to remain always a child. For what is the worth of human life, unless it is woven into the life of our ancestors by the records of history?" (Cicero, *Orator*, 46 BC).

Whipp goes on to talk about the anxiety some donor offspring feel about missing medical information and adds:

Our dissatisfaction has also been tempered with the knowledge that adoptees in the UK were given the right to access their birth records as long ago as the mid-1970s, yet no official records concerning donor conceptions have been maintained at all until the setting up of the HFEA in 1991. (Whipp 2004)

Unfortunately, many countries, including the United States, have been slow to react to these concerns. Barbara Sumner Burstyn summarizes these sentiments in her article "The new underclass" by stating:

...allowing technology to willfully create an underclass of people who are unaware of their genetic background and to support parents in denying their children their biological history is to continue the social, medical, and emotional disadvantages that have been suffered for generations by adopted people. (Burstyn 2004)

As the Donor Sibling Registry has grown and the need for it been expressed worldwide, founder Wendy Kramer has tried to use the media to familiarize the public with the needs and desires of some donor offspring to know where they came from and to whom they are connected. She has surveyed 751 offspring and found that although the vast majority are happy, well-functioning people, they have a need to know their genetic relatives. For some, it is simple curiosity: "Whom do I look like?" or "Where did this interest or talent come from?" For others, there is a need to know up-to-date medical information. Not surprisingly, many donor offspring become most curious around times of major life events such as marriage and becoming parents themselves.

Egg donation, together with other assisted reproductive technologies (ARTs), also directly led to the ability to evaluate embryos carefully and eliminate defective ones before they are transferred to the uterus. While this increases the chance that couples will have healthy babies, it has sparked the debate about creating "designer babies." Just how much say should individuals have about what type of baby should be created or destroyed? This illustrates two central ethical dilemmas: should people be allowed/encouraged to create "designer babies" and how can "fertility tourism" be regulated?

Questions arise also about the donors: as they prepare to donate, are they being adequately counseled on the potential long-term consequences of their donation? These include possible medical problems. In their 2009 paper "US oocyte donors: a retrospective study of medical and psychosocial issues," Kramer, Schneider and Schultz raise concerns about the risks of ovarian hyperstimulation, including future infertility and some evidence of increased risk of uterine, breast and other cancers. The 2011 film *Eggsploitation* sounds a louder alarm bell. It follows three former donors who encountered serious medical problems that they relate to egg donation. A common theme is that prospective donors are not adequately counseled about potential medical risks.

Another concern for donors is how they will feel about their offspring. Donor agency advertisements appeal to prospective donors by telling them of the happiness they will bring to people who want and deserve to be parents. What the ads do not focus on is what it will mean for these women—and their parents, siblings, children—to have genetic offspring that they do not know. I (Ellen) recently had a phone call from a woman who donated her eggs ten years ago "at a time when I was not thinking at all about having children" and who had recently been found by the recipient couple. The donor spent three "amazing" days with the family but returned home with unexpected feelings "that I can't begin to explain." She went on to say that everything seems different now that she is married and thinking about starting a family. More significant, she said she was "unprepared for the intense feelings of love" she has for the child she helped create.

Finally, the recipients. Egg donation has allowed older women, many of whom have entered menopause, to turn back their biological clocks and give birth. There are reports of women in their late 50s, even 60s, having babies. While this is still not a common occurrence, egg donation allows its possibility. This forces us to ask: is this a good thing? Some argue that if a woman in her 50s is married to a man in his 30s, why shouldn't they have a child together? Others support this option for a different reason: they say that age brings a wisdom and maturity that can be as valuable in parenting as youthfulness and energy. Either way, the question must be asked: is it fair to a young adult in his mid-20s to have a parent or parents in their late 70s?

Another ethical concern for recipients involves the promotion of anonymity. Until recently, donors and recipient women were often discouraged, sometimes even prevented, from meeting one another. Fortunately, as a result of increasing work with families doing open adoptions, awareness is growing of the potential benefits to the recipient, as well as to the donor and child, of meeting someone you will, in a sense, be connected to for life. It is increasingly common for donors and recipients to meet and to transform anonymous donation into a new form of known donation. These meetings may not include fully identifying information, but both donors and recipients proceed with egg donation aware that, in some ways, they will have a lifelong connection. In her article "Parents Anonymous" in *New Ways of Making Babies* Cynthia Cohen, writes:

> The special nature of this gift—assistance in bringing a child into being—obligates recipients to express their gratitude by viewing donors as more than anonymous surds. It obliges recipients to view them as actual, characterizable, morally considerable persons who are deserving of respect and appreciation. Donors are individuals whose needs, interests, and rights ought to be taken into account in the process of gamete donation. Givers also incur a moral obligation when they provide a gift—the obligation to give a complete gift and not just part of one. The gift that gamete donors give includes their genetic material. To complete this gift, donors must provide recipients, and ultimately the resulting children, with relevant information that may be carried with the genetic material. (Cohen 1996, p.95)

Who chooses egg donation?

Let's imagine that you are standing in the "departure lounge for egg donation."

It's a large, busy space, and you are, most likely, feeling somewhat bewildered. Whatever it is that brings you to consider egg donation, you are not where you once expected to be in your family-building journey. Yes, this departure lounge offers you hope and opportunity, but you are probably feeling a bit dazed. As you look around you at others considering egg donation, you will see a variety of people and a range of expressions on their faces. Some are weary travelers—they have been struggling to become parents for a long time, and their faces reveal the arduousness of their journey. Others look excited and energetic—perhaps this is their first departure lounge. Some women stand alone, some with their husbands or partners, and you may notice a few male couples, as they too have joined the ranks of those considering and pursuing egg donation.

In the pages that follow we will introduce the various situations that bring women and men to egg donation. We will also identify some of the specific questions and challenges that face each cohort of prospective egg donor parents. We hope that familiarizing you with fellow travelers will help ease your journey.

Primary ovarian insufficiency

Because women in their 20s and early 30s are assumed to have young, healthy eggs, most women in this age group do not anticipate infertility—at least not infertility due to egg quality. Sadly, there are young families who excitedly decide to have a baby only to learn that the woman has "bad eggs."

Because there has been no reason to assume an egg problem, some young women with poor egg quality try for years to conceive with no success. They may learn they have primary ovarian insufficiency (POI, which is sometimes also called premature ovarian failure, or POF, in cases where the ovary has stopped working completely) when a physician takes—and often retakes—a Day 3 FSH (follicle stimulating hormone) level, AMH (anti-mullerian hormone) levels or levels of other hormones such as estrogen. Together, these tests can provide an indication of a problem with egg quantity and/or quality.

As if it is not confusing enough, there are some women whose FSH and other levels appear to be normal but who, nonetheless, are probably infertile due to poor egg quality. These women are usually considered to have unexplained infertility until they undergo more extensive testing. To everyone's surprise, they are then found to be "poor responders." This unfortunate label refers to those women who, even when prescribed large amounts of potent ovulation-stimulating drugs, fail to produce more than a few follicles at best. However they come upon it, the diagnosis of poor ovarian reserve in a young woman is bewildering and often devastating. Women wonder how this could be, what they might have done to harm their eggs, why they had no warning of a problem. Indeed, they, like their fellow travelers, will learn, again and again, that reproduction is a mystery, but, at the time of diagnosis, it is only natural to look for answers, for causes, for blame and responsibility. Some will explore environmental factors, such as exposure to toxic chemicals, which can damage both eggs and sperm. Others will wonder about genetics. For example, I (Ellen) have a client, a young physician, who was found to have POI at age 33. When she discussed this with her mother, who had had her three children in her 20s, her mother remembered that she had begun to experience symptoms of menopause in her early 30s.

When a young woman under 40 learns that she has "old eggs," she faces several questions. The first is: is the condition permanent? While a 44-year-old woman with high FSH should be pretty certain that her egg supply is not going to be replenished, a young woman may wonder if the condition might reverse itself. Most reproductive endocrinologists have had a patient, here and there, who had elevated FSH, or otherwise documented poor ovarian quality, and who spontaneously became pregnant.

Despite discouraging FSH or AMH levels, a good egg happens along and is fertilized. Sadly, this is not the norm.

In addition to hoping for a spontaneous reversal and pregnancy, questions inevitably arise about what a woman might do to improve her egg quality. Since it is a mystery why she has diminished ovarian reserve, she must also wonder whether there is something she can do to give her a better chance of conceiving. Some women have turned to acupuncture, diet or herbal remedies in an effort to reinvigorate or regenerate their eggs. In the book *Inconceivable: A Woman's Triumph over Despair and Statistics* (2001), author Julia Indichova claims to have lowered her FSH through more holistic approaches. However, scientific evidence of women improving their egg quality through alternative therapies or diet is not well established.

The young women who come to the departure lounge for egg donation because they have "old eggs" may not be so quick to request egg donation. For one thing, they may need to take some time before they are really convinced that they can't use their own eggs. Some are hoping for a medical advance that will resolve their problem. Or they may simply want to wait a bit in the hope that they may be one of the lucky ones who find themselves unexpectedly pregnant.

There are other reasons for waiting. Cost is one. Egg donation is costly, and young couples are the least likely to have the savings at hand to pursue this option. For them, infertility is all the more devastating because it comes at a time when they are still launching their careers and perhaps saving for a house.

FXPOI

FXPOI (Fragile X-associated primary ovarian insufficiency) is a condition in which the ovaries are not functioning at full capacity in a woman who is an FMR1 premutation carrier, which is the gene that causes Fragile X syndrome—a genetic condition that causes intellectual disability, behavioral and learning challenges, and various physical characteristics. Common symptoms of FXPOI include absent or irregular periods, symptoms of menopause such as hot flashes and vaginal dryness, and infertility. For women who are diagnosed with POI, it is important to know if you also have an FMR1 premutation. If you have already been tested and are confirmed to be a FMR1 premutation carrier, there is about a 20–25 percent chance you will also experience POI. While many women with the FMR1 premutation can become pregnant, all carriers are at risk for having children with Fragile X syndrome so it is important to talk with a genetic counselor about your risk.

Declining ovarian reserve

There was a time, not all that long ago, when a woman giving birth after age 30 was labeled a "geriatric mother." In fact, there was a documentary in the 1970s called *Joyce at 34* (Chopra and Weill 1973). It was about a couple who decided—at the "old age of 34"—to have a baby. The film shows the couple announcing their "geriatric" pregnancy to Joyce's family, all of whom react with surprise and wonder.

The August 3, 2012, issue of the *New York Times Magazine* features an interview with then *Cosmopolitan* magazine's editor-in-chief, Kate White, in which she says:

> We ran an article that pained me to run, but I felt it was important. It basically said the key time to try to get pregnant is between 25 and 35. There has been so much said about still waiting until you're older, and I didn't have my first kid until I was 37, but we're taking a chance—you need to know it. (Zimmerman 2012)

The author (Edith Zimmerman) writes, "I asked her why it pained her." White offered the following response: "I want every girl to feel that she can have her first child at 50 if she wants."

Perspectives have changed and the popular media has played a big role in promoting these changed perspectives. White openly acknowledges the wish to let women think that they can have children at 50, but she also acknowledges that biology has not changed. The fact is that although many women want to become pregnant in their late 30s and early 40s, and shifting social norms support this, women's eggs still age at the same pace.

Although some women are able to conceive successful pregnancies with their own eggs into their early 40s, the fact remains that women experience declining fertility after age 35 and rapid drop-off after age 40.

Many women in the departure lounge of egg donation are in their late 30s and early 40s. They have come here from various places. Some have delayed childbearing while others have been struggling with infertility for a number of years. Along the way their eggs have aged and diminished ovarian reserve compounds their problems. Some were worried about fertility all along and had considered having a baby on their own or explored egg freezing. I (Ellen) recently had a client who was one of the first to electively freeze eggs five years ago. Sadly, when it came time to thaw them and attempt pregnancy, few survived the thaw and none of the resulting embryos led to an ongoing pregnancy.

Another group are women with secondary infertility. Some may have had a child or children years earlier and now find themselves wanting another. However they got here, women who arrive at the departure lounge of egg donation in their late 30s and early 40s feel they are racing against a biological clock that is ticking rapidly. Each month that passes weighs heavily upon them. They fear that the last good eggs are slipping away, and they worry that even if they do conceive, they will be prone to miscarriage. FSH numbers loom large, taking on a life and power of their own.

Women with diminished ovarian reserve are not in menopause. These are women whose egg quality is declining, but it is unlikely that all their "good" eggs are gone. While fertility starts to decrease significantly after the age of 35, it is impossible to predict exactly when this will happen for individual women or how long a woman's eggs will actually last. Hence they face a dilemma in considering egg donation: if they move forward and conceive with donated eggs, they may miss out on that one last opportunity to have a baby with their own eggs. Such "miracle" conceptions could occur with IVF or spontaneously. Some of these women face this dilemma and conclude that it is more important to have a baby now than to hold out for the off chance they will conceive and carry with their own eggs. Others decide to hold off on pursuing egg donation, feeling that they need to exhaust any possibility of using their own eggs.

Age-related infertility

Late marriages, second marriages, no marriages or occasionally the death of a child prompt women in their mid to late 40s or older to seek pregnancy. Unlike the women with diminished or diminishing ovarian reserve, these women know that their eggs are no longer viable. Although this awareness brings profound feelings of loss for some, many are also relieved to learn that there remains a way for them to be pregnant and, for those who have a male partner, to have their husband/partner's baby. They are happy to hear that their age does not adversely impact their chances of having a successful pregnancy with egg donation. It is true there are some pregnancy complications, such as pre-eclampsia and gestational diabetes that increase with age. However, older women who maintain a recommended body weight, are otherwise in good health and seek appropriate prenatal care should be able to anticipate healthy pregnancies.

Egg donation releases older women from the grip of the biological time clock. However, it does not free them from concerns about what it means to be older parents. Although they are youthful and energetic at 45 or 46, some are looking ahead and wondering how they will be at 68 or 70 when they have a child in college. They want to do right by their child and avoid being any older when their hoped-for child is born. For this reason, many choose to move as rapidly as they can with egg donation or to take a serious look at adoption.

Lost ovarian function due to surgery or illness

With advances in cancer treatment, increasing numbers of people are surviving at the expense of their fertility. Infertility after chemotherapy and/or radiation cannot always be accurately predicted. There are women who have aggressive treatment and who are later delighted to find that their menses return. They may go on to conceive and carry without difficulty. By contrast, there are others whose treatment damages their fertility. With chemotherapy, the common observation (a National Cancer Institute Alert, May 1988) has been that the greater the dose, the longer the duration of chemotherapy and the older the age of the woman at the time of treatment, the more likely the sacrifice of ovarian function.

The emerging field of "Oncofertility" is offering more options for both men and women facing cancer treatment. Increasingly, infertility clinics are developing programs to meet the needs of the ten percent of newly diagnosed cancer patients who are under the age of 45 (Rodrigues, Camp-Engelstein and Emanuel 2013). A woman likely to lose ovarian function may take a chance on egg freezing. If she is married or with a partner, she may undergo an IVF cycle, have her eggs inseminated with her husband or partner's sperm and cryopreserved for future use. In addition, there are newer and more experimental options such as whole ovary cryopreservation and the freezing of ovarian tissue. For boys younger than reproductive age, and thus unable to cryopreserve semen, an option being investigated includes freezing testicular tissue. Oncofertility is becoming increasingly important as more and more young people are surviving cancer and going on to live full lives that include building families.

Cancer is not the only medical problem that causes a woman to lose her ovaries and/or her ovarian function. A woman may have a cyst that ruptures and causes her to lose an ovary. Or a ruptured ectopic pregnancy may result in surgery in which she loses both ovary and fallopian tube. While most women have two ovaries and one may remain after a medical and surgical emergency, there are instances in which a woman loses both ovaries.

Egg donation after surgery, chemotherapy or radiation is attractive to some women, but not to others. Those who find it most attractive tend to focus on its restorative capacity: here is a woman who has lost half of her reproductive function and who can now use the remaining half—her ability to carry—to bring a new life into the world. For a woman who has been ill, and who probably confronted her own mortality, the opportunity to plant two (or more) new feet on this earth is profoundly moving.

Why, then, would some survivors of illness or surgery be reluctant to pursue egg donation? Some say that it brings back painful memories of the illness that robbed them of their fertility. Until they face their desire to have a family, they had been moving on in their lives, moving away from the cancer. The prospect of being back in a medical setting, of having invasive tests and procedures and of having the constant reminder of their battle with cancer is painful. Others may avoid egg donation because they fear the reactions they may see or perceive in others. What if the physician suggests a delay of a year or two or three before pregnancy? This could frighten a woman into fearing that her physician is waiting to see if she will have a recurrence. Cancer survivors need to believe in their own futures and, for the most part, feel confident that others do as well.

Women born without ovaries or without ovarian function
Sometimes women are born without ovaries or without the capacity to produce eggs. We can easily imagine what the opportunity to carry a baby must mean to these women. In this regard, they may be traveling lighter than others considering egg donation. Although some will choose adoption, many will regard egg donation as a gift, one that enables them to use another part of their reproductive function. As we mentioned, women in this situation may face fewer decisions than those with other reasons for considering egg donation. These women know that they will not be creating a full biological child. The opportunity to become pregnant and to have a child connected genetically to their partner and gestationally to themselves is inviting.

Unexplained infertility

In a time of advances in reproductive technology, unexplained infertility has to be one of the most baffling experiences. How is it that a couple can go to a skilled reproductive endocrinologist and be told there is no identifiable fertility problem? Worse still, they can seek a second and even third opinion and hear the same thing again and again: "Something is wrong but we don't know what it is."

Not long ago, couples were labeled "normal infertile." How bad was that? Bad enough to prompt people to feel that their problems must be psychological. After all, if there was no apparent physical problem, they must be causing their own infertility with ambivalent thoughts, bad behavior, past misdeeds or some other curse.

Families struggling with unexplained infertility find themselves in the world of trial and error. With little to go by, physicians suggest trying IVF, hoping that the explanation of the infertility rests in the way that the egg is released (or not released) or in difficulties that egg and sperm have when they encounter each other. For some people with unexplained infertility, IVF provides a solution. But what of others? What do you do if your infertility remains all the more unexplained after repeated failed IVF attempts?

Some couples with unexplained infertility consider egg and/or sperm donation, assuming that there must be some defect in their gametes, or they may wonder, sadly, if the "mix" between them doesn't work. Some with unexplained infertility who turn to egg donation still do not become pregnant. What then? One such couple tried donor sperm and, eventually, a gestational carrier before deciding to adopt. Another tried a second egg donor, conceived and enjoyed a successful pregnancy. Still another moved on to embryo placement and had not one but two successful pregnancies. Another option is to continue trying on their own, knowing that some couples with unexplained fertility have spontaneous pregnancies.

Genetic issues

Some people learn, through genetic testing before a pregnancy is attempted, during a pregnancy or after a baby is born, that they are carriers of a serious, even lethal, genetic disorder. They may have close family members whom they have watched suffer from a genetic disorder. Some of these families have a baby die in utero. Some choose to terminate pregnancies when such a disorder is diagnosed in utero. Others deliver a child who dies at birth or soon after. Still others parent children with very challenging conditions. Veterans of each of these experiences may turn to egg or sperm donation in an effort to avoid transmitting the genetic abnormality to future pregnancies.

Preimplantation genetic diagnosis has enabled many families with genetic issues to avoid transmitting them to their offspring. Still, there remain some who turn instead to egg donation. These include women who have diminished ovarian reserve in addition to a genetic issue.

Women who can neither provide eggs nor carry a baby

Sometimes families must face more than one reproductive challenge in their journey to have a baby. Sometimes it is the woman who is hit with this double blow: she can neither produce viable eggs nor carry a successful pregnancy. In some instances, this is something a woman learns early in life and which a couple knows as they enter into marriage and make plans to build a family. In other instances, the double blow unfolds sequentially. A woman undergoing a fertility work-up may be advised that she has a uterine abnormality and later learn she has elevated FSH. Or she may have turned to egg donation and later learns, through a failed cycle of further medical exploration, that she also has uterine abnormalities.

The decision to use both donor eggs and a gestational carrier is very different for those who know from the start and those who learn along the way. Couples who know from the start face one decision: "Do we want to turn to two women to help us bring a child into this world that has a genetic connection to one of us and a parenting bond with both of us or do we want to adopt?" Couples who learn along the way face a two-part decision. For them, one decision is made. Only after they are comfortable with it and accustomed to it do they face a second decision. As one woman who is now the mother of three children, all through a combination of egg donation and a gestational carrier, said:

> For us it was a decision made in steps. We ended up doing something we never, ever thought we would do. That is because our reality changed along the way. This experience taught us an important lesson: "Never say never." It taught us to be much more open-minded.

Families choosing to have a child through egg donation and gestational care face several issues. One is ethical. Is it morally and ethically correct to bring a child into this world when he will have neither a genetic nor a gestational connection to his mother? A second issue is logistical. It is complicated enough to embark upon either an egg donor or a gestational carrier pregnancy; combining the two involves a great deal of medical, psychological and legal coordination. Then there are financial challenges. This is undoubtedly a very costly venture—often upwards of $80,000 simply for the chance of conception. Finally, there is the question of what to do if the gestational carrier does not become pregnant. With so many variables, it is difficult to know which one to address. Families and their physicians wonder if they should try a second time with the same participants and same protocol, change the protocol, change the egg donor or, perhaps, the gestational carrier?

Single women

Look around any fertility center waiting room and there are single women who have decided to try to have a baby before it is too late. Most started with simple donor inseminations, but as they work their way up the fertility center food chain, they often find themselves all the way at IVF. And if that doesn't work, then what?

Some single women who have already made the decision to use sperm donation unexpectedly find themselves considering egg donation as well. Some do so because they feel so strongly about being pregnant and having a gestational connection to their child. Others turn to egg donation because they know that it is often difficult for a single woman to adopt. Many will say, "I feel I have more control this way than with adoption."

An additional ethical issue arises with single women. Is it fair to intentionally create a child who will have only one parent? This question becomes all the more poignant when the intended parent is older. Add to that the fact that the one parent is not the child's genetic mother. Going through this list, it becomes easy to see why many would say, "Stop. This is too much. Reproductive medicine has gone too far when it creates a child who will not be parented by either of his genetic parents, will have only one parent and that parent will be of advanced age." Everything might seem clear in the abstract, but not always so much when there are real people.

Meet Jenny

Jenny is a 47-year-old physician and the over-the-top-in-love mother of Olivia, now nearly two. Like so many women who eventually turn to egg donation, Jenny wanted to be a mom for most of her life. When she found herself still single in her early 40s, Jenny briefly considered having a child on her own.

Then came Pierre. Pierre, three years her junior, was the love of Jenny's life. She met him through friends and they were engaged within a few weeks and married in six months. Jenny and Pierre began trying to conceive before their marriage and went right to treatment after a few months of trying. Even with the invasive tests and procedures, they were blissfully happy and totally delighting in finally having lasting love.

But it was not meant to be. Pierre was not feeling well, lost some weight inexplicably and complained of a strange itching feeling. Jenny pushed him to see his doctor who was initially reassuring but soon suspected that Pierre had leukaemia. Although aggressive chemotherapy seemed to be working, Pierre succumbed to the disease barely two years after he and Jenny were married. He left

Jenny with several vials of frozen semen which he had frozen upon diagnosis.

Jenny was 44 when Pierre died. She allowed herself several months to grieve but then began thinking, perhaps more intensely than ever, about pregnancy. Jenny questioned whether it was wise for her to embark upon single motherhood in her mid-40s but felt more optimistic when her younger brother and his wife, parents of three children themselves, were supportive of the idea. Their offer to be guardians of a child further bolstered Jenny's confidence. She consulted her doctor about using Pierre's frozen semen and was told, "Your eggs are old now. It's a real long shot, but you have nothing to lose by trying."

Jenny saw it differently. She did have something to lose. Something big—Pierre's sperm. For her it was more important for her to have Pierre's baby than one conceived with her eggs. Although her doctor and others offered little support for the idea, Jenny began looking for an egg donor. When she found her, their collaborative efforts brought Olivia into the world.

Male couples

It is no longer unusual to find two men sitting together in the waiting room of a reproductive medicine clinic. Eager to have children together and often discouraged from adoption, a number of pioneering gay couples have turned to egg donation with a gestational carrier. Theirs is a very complicated and costly path to parenthood, but one that affords them the opportunity to share in a pregnancy, to lovingly create a child and to have a child with a biological connection to one of them.

Since two men intending to have a child together know for certain that they need eggs, they confront none of the "what if" questions that many heterosexual couples face. There is simply no question of trying another medication protocol or seeing another physician as a means of attaining better egg quality. Hence, gay couples, for all the challenges they face, are at least spared the question "Do we really need an egg donor?" They do.

Gay couples must also decide who will provide the genetic material. "Do we want to have one of us be the biological father and have the other partner's sister donate eggs?" If so, then there does, of course, need to be a sister who is ready, willing and able to donate. What if there are two sisters? What if both offer to donate? What if neither offers? Do we ask? What if each man has a sister or close friend and both are willing to donate? In order to maximize their chances of having a baby, a gay couple might find themselves trying to figure out who is likely to be most fertile. It's easy to see how this could all become very complicated, very fast! That said, increasing numbers of gay couples are making their way successfully through a maze of decisions and a mountain of costs and becoming parents with the help of egg donation.

Female couples

Perhaps it seems odd to think that couples consisting of two women might find themselves in the departure lounge of egg donation. After all, as one lesbian woman said to me (Ellen), "You'd think that with four ovaries we'd have some good eggs." However, infertility does not discriminate and even lesbian couples can encounter egg problems.

Female couples also turn to egg donation for reasons other than infertility in both of them. For legal reasons and for parity, some lesbian couples decide that one will donate her eggs to the other, who will carry their baby. Hence, each becomes an equal player—legally and emotionally—in creating their child. In some instances, there may be medical reasons for the donation: the partner desirous of pregnancy may not be the one with "good eggs," allowing her partner to be the donor. Or the couple may simple prefer to conceive this way if one woman prefers to be pregnant and the other to pass on her generic heritage. I (Ellen) know one such couple in which the Vietnamese-born partner wanted to pass on her cultural heritage and her American-born, Caucasian partner wanted to be pregnant.

To state the obvious, lesbian couples require sperm donors. Hence, those who are also pursuing egg donation travel down a path that is complicated medically and logistically. It is also expensive and, in many ways, emotionally uncharted. Sometimes the woman who ends up carrying the baby is not the partner who really cared—at the beginning—about being pregnant. Sometimes the one donating her eggs didn't care as much about a genetic connection as a gestational one.

As we have seen throughout this chapter, people enter the departure lounge of egg donation for a variety of reasons. Many of our travelers carry a heavy load. They are women who have wanted to become mothers for years and, for one reason or another, time has run out (or is running out) on their eggs. Others travel somewhat lightly. They may have had children years ago and now, much older and in a second marriage, feel grateful that there is way that they can still bear a child. Male couples probably feel overwhelmed by costs and the complexity of the process but appreciate finally having a place in any departure lounge for parenthood.

Some of our travelers will spend time in the departure lounge of egg donation but ultimately decide to take a different course to parenthood. Others will acquaint themselves with egg donation and feel fortified to pursue it. In the next chapter we will take a look at the ways in which people approach egg donation, at the questions you are likely to ask yourselves and at some of the answers you may find.

– 3 –
Deciding Whether to Pursue Egg Donation

Here you are at a crossroads in your journey toward parenthood. You can either travel down the road of egg donation or you can choose another path. Before you focus on whether or not to use donated eggs, we encourage you to pause and consider all of the choices that lie before you. Since most of you will be traveling as part of a couple, we encourage each of you to turn to your companion in this journey and to remind yourselves that you must come to decisions that will work for both of you and for your relationship.

Elements of decision making

Like all travelers, you should plan well for the journey. We'd like to begin by reminding you of some of the elements of and influences on decision making that we addressed in Chapter 2 and then offer additional suggestions.

Decisions are made sequentially

If you have been struggling with infertility, you have probably already figured out that as your reality changes, so do your perceptions of your options. How many of you once thought, "I'll never do IVF?" By now, many of you are veterans of IVF cycles many times over. As you traveled down one path, you discovered that options which once seemed disturbing have actually become attractive.

Never say never

You have probably figured this out as well. It is easy to say you will never do this or never do that, but, as we said before, as your reality changes, so do your decisions. Remember also, that "not yet" does not mean "never." For instance, your partner may say "not yet" to something that you think you want to do. Listen carefully and remember: "Not yet is not never."

Husbands and wives move at different paces and this is not necessarily a bad thing

Remember that we said, "Not yet is not never." If you are like most couples facing decisions about using donated eggs, one of you will be ready to consider this option before the other. When this happens, the person who wants to move forward is often upset and angry with the one who says, "I'm not ready" or "We need to try...again."

Are you puzzled when we say that this is not necessarily a bad thing? In fact, we have found that couples have a way of balancing each other. One of you can sound—and feel—eager to explore options beyond conventional treatment, in part because you know that your partner will slow you down and help ensure that you make wise, informed decisions. Similarly, you who are trailing at the rear can afford to take it slowly because you trust your spouse to take the lead.

Your history will inform your decision making

Decisions about choosing egg donation, adoption and other options will be shaped by your past experiences. If your favorite cousins were adopted, you will have one set of associations about adoption. If you were a birth mother and placed a child in adoption, your feelings about adoption will be influenced by this experience, and if your cousin's daughter was an egg donor, you will have her as a reference point for egg donation. Your losses also will help shape your perceptions of each of these options. Which leads us to…

Loss and grief are part of the journey

Be prepared for a journey—or the continuation of a journey—that involves loss and grief and ever-unfolding new realities. We hope that you, like others who have traveled before you, will discover the unanticipated rewards that come from being able to accept loss, to grieve and then to celebrate your new realities.

Infertility researcher Dr. Stacy Ellender captures this in an essay she wrote about her own infertility experience and her daughter's arrival from China in *Experiencing Infertility*. She writes:

> Someday, my daughter will learn that she was "forsaken on the street," abandoned under unknown circumstances, and waves of pain may send her reeling. But I like to think that I will steady her, that we will share our stories of loss and redefinition. I can hold her hand in mine and show her how to face pain with honesty, integrity and a deep wonder at its unexpected potential to shape our lives. (Ellender 1998, p.268)

Don't punish yourselves

Remember that you have made the best decisions you could along the way. Regret is a poisonous feeling, and infertile people are often the maestros of regret. It is so tempting to look back and second-guess yourself. "I should have been less focused on my career and we should have tried earlier." "I shouldn't have had an abortion when I was 22. It might have been my only chance to have a baby." "I should have pushed my husband when he said we had time to wait." "I should have met him earlier."

It is almost inevitable that you will look back and contemplate how things could have been different if only you had made different choices. Try to be gentle with yourselves and each other and remember you did the best you could with the information you had at hand.

The people you meet along the way will shape your journey

People struggling with infertility find one another in doctors' waiting rooms and online through sites and support groups.

These resources often become all the more important when you are considering egg donation or adoption or surrogacy. Finding fellow travelers reminds you that you are not alone. Hearing from those who have traveled the path before you can be even more valuable. Nothing is as reassuring as to hear from others who took alternative paths and reached happy endings.

The people you meet along your journey will have a lot to do with the choices you make. This is, for the most part, a good thing. We expect that you will find mentors and friends. But exercise caution as well. You are vulnerable. You will be listening carefully and with emotion to everything you hear about the options that lie before you. If someone has had a bad story using an option that you are considering, that doesn't mean that everyone's experience is bad or that yours will be.

You will meet people along the way who will become friends for the journey. You may also meet people who will become friends for life.

You have the right to make your own decisions and to feel that you are doing so free and clear of the influence of others

As you travel this journey, you will surely find that others will offer advice. First of all, you will receive a tremendous amount of medical information. You should take all of this information in and consider it carefully before making your own decision. Be prepared for medical professionals to know more about egg donation than adoption—many are likely to favor it as an option.

You will receive additional advice from what we call "the self-appointed experts"—the family members, friends and complete strangers who want to give you such sage advice as, "Relax and you will get pregnant" or "Parenthood is not so great anyhow" or "Why don't you just adopt?" You will need to remain strong and sure-footed as this advice comes your way, often when you feel least equipped to cope with it.

Speak from a position of strength

Do not tempt advice givers! If you let people know only the basic facts about your situation—that you want to have a baby and that you are doing your best to make that happen—you are less likely to invite unsolicited advice. And this is really all that anyone needs to know.

When you do have some news that you want to share, speak from a position of strength. If you say, "We're thinking about using a donated egg" or "We are looking into adoption" you may get upsetting responses such as "Oh, we're so sorry IVF didn't work for you" or "Are you sure you've seen a good doctor? We know someone who had 25 miscarriages and then saw Dr. So-and-So in North Rural, South Dakota and..." or "Be careful, you know birth parents often decide to keep their babies."

What you need to say—if and when you say anything at all—is "We have *great* news. We've decided to..." or, better yet, "We have great news, we're expecting a child through..."

Assessing whether you can use your own eggs

A key milestone in deciding to try egg donation is concluding that it is unwise to try—or continue to try—with your own eggs. Short of a genetic disorder or the absence of ovaries, what proof does a couple have that donor eggs are needed?

Unfortunately, there is no test that can perfectly predict a woman's ability to become pregnant with her own eggs, so we will discuss some of the tools that physicians and nurses use to assess what is known as "ovarian reserve."

Nurse practitioner Carol Lesser of Boston IVF in Brookline, Massachusetts, works with many women in their early 40s seeking pregnancy. She notes that they are, for the most part, a youthful, energetic, optimistic group who had looked forward for many years to having children. Sadly, many are filled with regret and anger when they learn that their chances for having children using their own eggs are slim. "They are angry at themselves for delaying parenting, and they are angry at physicians for never warning them of the natural hazards of aging."

Lesser has found that, before she can offer medical guidance, she must help her patients with their feelings of anger and regret. She begins by assuring them that they have not done something wrong and explains that the ovary ages more rapidly than any other organ in the human body, and that by the time a woman reaches age 43, approximately 85 percent of her eggs are abnormal, regardless of her FSH.

With over 25 years of experience in the field of reproductive medicine, Lesser acknowledges that it was not until recently that obstetricians and gynecologists fully appreciated the impact of age on reproductive ability:

> Society has changed, but biology has not. In the past, when people did not live as long, a woman who completed her childbearing by age 30 or so was able to raise her children to adulthood. It made sense from an evolutionary standpoint. Today people are living longer and often preferring to have children later in life, but our ovaries are aging just as rapidly as they did a century ago. It is often very hard for women to accept this.

With no perfect, predictive test of ovarian function, how can a woman assess her chances of pregnancy with her own eggs? In addition to paying attention to chronological age, she can turn to the Day 3 FSH test, the most common measure of ovarian reserve (FSH is follicle stimulating hormone). Typically, on the second, third or fourth day of a woman's menstrual cycle, blood is drawn to measure FSH. Because testing for FSH varies from state to state, clinic to clinic and lab to lab, we cannot offer a universal guide for FSH results. However, a relatively low number is desired and a high number suggests decreased ovarian reserve, with sustained high levels seen in menopause. For example, many clinics hope that their patients will have Day 3 FSH numbers under 10, will interpret numbers between 10 and 15 as borderline, and will see numbers over 15 as worrisome. So, you might conclude, "If my FSH is low, my eggs should be fine."

If only it were that simple! FSH measures ovarian reserve, or the number of good-quality eggs that a woman has left. For some women, quantity is related to quality; for others, it is not.

Hence, it is possible for a woman to have a higher FSH, indicating fewer eggs, but still have some very good-quality eggs remaining. In addition, as women age, their Day 2, 3, or 4 estradiol level (estrogen) may be elevated at times. Estrogen suppresses FSH, so FSH levels are best interpreted in the presence of a normal estradiol level for more accuracy.

There are other tests of ovarian reserve. Many centers rely on an antral follicle assessment of a woman's ovaries, providing yet another measure of ovarian reserve. This test requires a vaginal ultrasound by a trained sonographer, and is often performed on Day 2, 3 or 4 of a woman's cycle, but can also be done at other times or while on oral contraceptives. Antral follicles are small potential egg sacs. Ovaries that have few or no antral follicles at the start of a woman's cycle will not respond well to many fertility medications and so may not be good IVF candidates. By contrast, those with a number of antral follicles are likely to produce the excess follicles that are desired in an IVF cycle.

Some physicians employ the clomiphene citrate challenge test, a test considered by some to be more precise than the simpler Day 3 FSH test. With the clomiphene citrate challenge test, a Day 3 FSH and estradiol level is obtained. If the level is reassuring, then the woman is prescribed 100mg of clomiphene citrate for five days early in a woman's cycle (usually Days 5 through 9). Her FSH is again measured on Day 10. Optimal results show FSH dropping on Day 10—or at least not rising significantly. Conversely, if it rises at that point, it is thought to indicate diminished ovarian reserve. Estradiol is also measured on Day 3.

The newest and most promising blood test measures AMH (anti-mullerian hormone). This test is gaining in popularity because it is the first blood marker to both predict and assess a woman's ovarian reserve. In other words, studies are showing that when an AMH level is obtained in younger women, the higher the number, the less concern there is for premature ovarian insufficiency or failure. In contrast to FSH levels, a higher AMH is reassuring. The result can help predict who will be a good candidate for fertility medications and IVF and who will not be. It is also used to assess whether a potential egg donor would be a good candidate for donation.

Carol Lesser reminds women that chronological age is as—or more—important as ovarian age and test results. She notes that women with advanced ovarian and chronological age generally have a lower chance of a successful pregnancy using their own eggs than either younger women or women with "younger" ovarian age. It is also possible for a woman to have eggs that are plentiful, look good and fertilize well, but which, when fertilized, still do not create a healthy embryo. The most likely reason for this is again maternal age.

So what does all of this have to do with the fork in the road? A lot. Inevitably, there are some women who have elevated FSH who will conceive. Similarly, there are women 43 and 44 who will succeed in becoming pregnant and who will give birth at an age at which some women are already grandmothers. How, then, do those of you who are at the fork in the road decide between trying on your own, with or without IVF, and using donor eggs? A first step is to consider carefully how important it is to you at this point to have a genetic connection to your child. You should look at this question in light of your age, your stamina, your financial resources and the impact that prolonged treatment is having on your marriage and other relationships.

For those for whom using their own genetic material remains a high priority, we want to offer some brief discussion of two treatment options that could result in the birth of a couple's full biological child.

Continuing to try on your own (without IVF)

Some women are not ready to give up on the possibility of having a child with their own eggs, but they choose to try on their own rather than with IVF. What distinguishes this group from those who try IVF—or more IVF—before taking the egg donation fork in the road? Financial cost is a significant factor for many, but there are other issues as well. The most important involves determining if IVF offers any benefit over trying naturally. Surely it does when a woman has blocked tubes or there is a severe male factor, but what of the couple considering egg donation only because of egg quality?

Carol Lesser observes that the higher the FSH, the less treatment matters. She explains that if a woman has a low FSH, she is likely to have many eggs. Even if most of the eggs are flawed, some good ones should remain. IVF, with its controlled hyperstimulation and retrieval of eggs, enables the physician to go after a large group of eggs all at once. It is hoped that this large group will contain at least one egg of good quality. Perhaps two or three will fertilize, and if all are transferred, the result may be an ongoing pregnancy. Lesser's point is that, by doing IVF, someone with a large number of eggs but declining fertility is able to condense several natural cycles into one month.

Without adequate ovarian reserve, women are less likely to benefit from IVF. There aren't as many eggs to begin with, and so an IVF cycle is unlikely to yield the quantity of eggs that would increase the odds of a successful pregnancy. Lesser and many others have observed that women with high FSH who become pregnant often do so on their own spontaneously, unless, of course, blocked tubes or severe male factor renders this impossible.

Trying on your own, without IVF, before choosing egg donation, offers a number of benefits, assuming a couple can afford for time to pass. For one thing, there is the emotional benefit of having some time to transition to egg donation and to do so feeling certain that you are not going to succeed with your own eggs. In addition, there is that matter of the "lucky egg." If a lucky egg is going to come along, you can't be pregnant with a donated egg. So those who hold out some hope that they will conceive on their own benefit from delaying an egg donation pregnancy.

Some women attempt to lower their FSH level. There are many anecdotal stories of success with acupuncture, as well as with herbal supplements or special diets, including one that recommends eating large amounts of wheat grass, weekly acupuncture and meditation. It is difficult to assess whether or not any of these approaches could actually make a difference, since there are natural fluctuations in FSH and pregnancies can occur in a few instances with elevated FSH levels. What we do know is that trying alternative approaches such as acupuncture can help you to feel better. Many women report a generalized sense of well-being and, in the face of a dreadful sense of helplessness, they are grateful to be able to do something that feels proactive.

Another reason for trying on one's own comes back to that thorny issue of regret. If you have struggled with infertility for any time at all, you probably know that regret is the most painful of emotions. Some couples decide to try for a time on their own because they want to avoid looking back and wondering, "Could we have done it on our own if we'd been more patient?"

Finally, trying on one's own buys time. It buys time to save money for egg donation or for adoption. It buys time possibly to benefit from medical advances. It buys time for a woman to grieve not being able to pass on some special part of herself and time for her partner to grieve this loss as well. It allows a couple to grieve the fact that fertility treatments did not work for them, to regroup and replenish their relationship, to feel that, when they get to the next fork in the road, they will be all the better prepared to make the best decision for themselves.

Continuing to try with IVF

And, for those still hopeful of using their own eggs, there also remains the option of moving to IVF (or, for many reading this book, continuing with IVF treatments for a while longer).

In vitro fertilization refers to fertilization outside the human body. In regular IVF a woman takes medication that causes her to produce several ovarian follicles. Follicular growth is carefully monitored by ultrasound, as well as by blood tests. When a number of follicles have grown beyond 15 centimeters, eggs are retrieved in what is a minor surgical procedure. They are then mixed with the intended father's sperm, placed in a special culture medium for two to five days and then transferred back to the intended mother's uterus via a catheter. Regular IVF differs from donor-IVF in that it is the intended mother's own eggs, rather than those of a donor, that are fertilized and transferred to her.

Costs for IVF vary worldwide, as does insurance coverage and government mandates for treatment. If you are considering trying/continuing IVF with your own eggs, it is important to determine the financial costs and assess whether you can afford them. The website **www.ivfcost.net** offers helpful explanations of costs as well as useful charts that consider costs in light of success rates. For example, the average cost in 2010 for one cycle of IVF in the United States was about $12,000, while in Italy it was about $5500. However, most intended parents require more than one cycle to achieve success. Also, additional procedures such as ICSI (intracytoplasmic sperm injection), assisted hatching and PGD (preimplantation genetic diagnosis) are not usually included.

Depending upon whether you live where IVF costs are covered by insurance or are less expensive and depending upon your personal finances, the decision to try—or continue to try— regular IVF or to turn to egg donation may be driven by the costs involved.

In addition to looking at your finances, you should pay attention to the potential toll that continued IVF takes on your marriage, relationships with family and friends, and career, as well as the cost of further delaying parenthood.

Your next steps

Since this is a book about egg donation, we assume that, for many of our readers, the next step after trying with your own eggs will be egg donation. However, we believe that part of making an informed decision about egg donation involves at least briefly considering other options, including other third-party parenting options, adoption and moving forward with the family you have.

In order to make a decision that will be best for you, it makes sense to look at why it is you want to have a child.

Exploring your motivations for parenthood

How and why does anyone decide to become a parent? If we were to pose that question to one of your fertile friends, they might respond, "I didn't think about it very much—I just knew I wanted to be a mom" or "It was just the natural order of things— you get married, buy a house, have a kid…" or "I love little babies and couldn't wait to have one to take care of."

We could add to the list, but, instead, we hope that you see our point: people who conceive easily may not give a lot of thought to what it means to be a parent. In addition, they are never called upon to consider the relative significance of different aspects of parenthood—how important it is to them to share a pregnancy experience, to have a genetic connection with their child or to continue a bloodline. They don't have to consider the impact of having their bodies and their sex lives invaded by a team of helpers in order to become parents. They don't have to ask themselves what it would mean to parent a child of another race or a child who was half genetically theirs or perhaps was their full genetic child gestated by another woman.

Although there are no easy answers to the multitude of questions you will ask yourself, there are some things that you can begin to do to help you to see things more clearly. We propose that you begin by asking yourselves the following questions.

1. *Why do you want to be a parent?* How many of your responses have to do with having a physical connection to the child—genetic or gestational? How many have to do with your expectations and dreams about the parenting role and experience? If you have a parenting partner, how many have to do with the notion of blending your genes with your beloved's to create a child to parent together?

2. *What does it mean to be a member of your family?* Is your family one in which there has been intermarriage— religious or racial? Is your family one with a strong ethnic or cultural identity? Is it one that celebrates diversity? Do you

have nieces and nephews who are of a different race to you, either because of adoption or transracial marriage?

3. *What are your beliefs about nature and nurture?* Are you someone who feels that people are molded by their genes or do you put stock in environmental influences? Where do your views on nature and nurture come from? Are they fixed or are you curious about other perspectives? Throughout this book we will encourage people to learn about epigenetics, the science of changes in the pattern of gene activity.

4. *What is it about parenthood that you look forward to?* When you picture yourself with a child, is it important that the child look like you? Do you imagine the child being like you in other ways that you perceive to be genetic?

In thinking through these questions, you will gain information that will help you make choices. For example, if genetic connection ranks high with you, adoption may move lower on your list of options—at least for now. If the actual experience of being a parent is the most important thing to the two of you, you may be willing to forgo the physical, emotional and financial risks of other options and plunge straight into adoption.

Comparing other options to egg donation

So here you are at a fork in the road. One path leads to egg donation. The other fork sends you down a different path—at least for the time being. As you face this next decision, remember that your perspective may change as your reality changes. You may travel down one path only to reach another fork in the road and the need for a different decision. But here you are at this fork. Let's take a look at the decisions you face and at the choices you see before you.

Embryo placement versus egg donation

In the earliest years of the 21st century, a new path to parenthood became available: embryo placement. This is often referred to as either *embryo donation* or *embryo adoption*. We are not comfortable with either term since *embryo donation* does not acknowledge the adoption-like aspects of this option, and *embryo adoption* is problematic for other reasons discussed below. We are most comfortable with *embryo placement*.

Embryo placement became an option because there are couples who go through IVF and cryopreserve or freeze embryos for possible future use and then, for a variety reasons, do not seek pregnancy with their cryopreserved embryos. This may happen when embryos remain after the couple has twins or triplets on the first IVF cycle, or has a second or third successful pregnancy using some cryopreserved embryos, or decides, for other reasons, including divorce and death, not to use the remaining embryos.

For some parents who were assisted by IVF, having extra embryos does not pose a problem, either emotionally or ethically. They see their embryos as having potential for life and feel they are fundamentally different from fetuses. Such couples generally feel comfortable either discarding extra embryos or donating them to science.

Some couples who go through IVF end up with embryos that they are prepared neither to parent nor to discard or donate to science. Included in this group are those who believe that life begins with an embryo and who are aware, as they enter into an IVF cycle, that the process may leave them seeking a home for their embryos.

There are others who enter a cycle with no particular concerns about their embryos but who later find themselves in a very painful predicament. This happens to some who feel so barren that they cannot imagine having more embryos than they are prepared to parent, as well as to those who discover, in the course of the IVF process or after having children, that their feelings about the origins of life have changed.

Psychologist Maggie Kirkman, senior research fellow at the Jean Halles Research Unit, School of Public Health and Preventative Medicine, Monash University, Australia, interviewed women who decided for and against embryo placement. She notes that it is the maternal feelings that some mothers feel towards their embryos that prompts them to donate them to another couple. Kirkman quotes Wilma, who considered reasons for and against donating and concluded, "One embryo became our second child, who is absolutely wonderful. Who were the others? Just as wonderful? They at least deserved a chance at life." Kirkman says:

> This sense of "child of ours" was marked in embryo donors and others who had contemplated embryo placement. It could be explained in terms of pre-implantation parental feelings known to be experienced by people undergoing IVF who look through a microscope at the dividing cells of their potential children. (Kirkman 2003b, p.2234)

However they get there, couples who have additional embryos and who believe that life begins with an embryo, not with a beating heart, are in a very difficult predicament: they feel they must find parents for their embryos. Until a few years ago they were left to try to resolve this dilemma on their own. Ironically, some felt they had to attempt a pregnancy they didn't want or they had to find women who wanted to become pregnant with placed embryos.

As adoption agencies became aware of the dilemma of couples with extra embryos, some stepped in and began to formalize and facilitate a process they termed *embryo adoption*. We feel it is important to remember the differences between traditional adoption, which involves finding a home for a baby or child that needs one, and embryo placement. In an article in *The Boston Globe* (2005), reproductive lawyer Susan Crockin writes:

> IVF patients have always had the option, among others, to donate their embryos to other patients, whether through their IVF clinics or through private agencies or programs with a wide variety of philosophical and religious perspectives. To force adoption frameworks onto cryopreserved embryos as a matter of law and

policy would significantly reduce those choices, while elevating one religious doctrine—that of the Christian right—over others. Changing the vocabulary to blur the distinction between four- to eight-cell embryos and born children—by naively or intentionally using terms like "embryo adoption," "preborn children," or "microscopic Americans" and those who create them "parents"—is not only legally wrong, but for those of us post-born people who value real adoption, choice, reproductive health, and stem cell research, bad public policy. Beware of agendas that may be lurking in the petri dish. (Crockin 2005)

Kansas based social worker, Kris Probasco, has an active practice of embryo placement. Probasco notes that while pregnancy through a placed embryo is not right for everyone, it offers some advantages to those who are otherwise considering egg donation and/or adoption. It is less costly than either of these options, since the embryos already exist and the donors are not seeking payment for them. For those who have faced disappointments in either egg donation or adoption, embryo placement can give them a head start—the embryo already exists and, once placed, it is theirs. Hence they are spared the disappointment that comes if a donor does not produce eggs or if an adoption falls through. Finally, for some, embryo placement seems morally more acceptable: conception has already occurred and the hoped-for child will be gestated by his/her parents.

Probasco supports her couples in many ways through the embryo placement process, facilitating meetings between donors and recipients, and helping recipients distinguish between emotional conception and physical conceptions. As she puts it, "The parents are the 'creators of their family.' They received help from another family." Probasco also helps the families maintain open relationships that benefit all their offspring.

If you are considering embryo placement, here are some things to consider.

THE CHILD'S STORY

As you begin to think about embryo placement, remember that children who enter their families through this process will have genetic families with full biological siblings being raised by the people who originally created them. Although some may be raised in open relationships such as those Probasco assists with, some embryo-placed offspring will grow up without contact with their biological siblings. Rather, they will grow up knowing that their full biological siblings were given the opportunity to be raised by their genetic parents but that they—because of a decision made by their parents, their parents' physicians and embryologists—must grow up without a genetic connection to their parents. As they mature, they may grapple with the knowledge that it probably took a split second for the embryologist to decide which embryos to transfer to the genetic parents and which to cryopreserve for some other future.

The story of a child created through embryo placement is similar to, and yet fundamentally different from, the story of the traditional adoptee. The traditional adoptee may also have full siblings being raised by his birth parents, but what he knows, painful as it may be to accept, is that, at the time of his birth, his parents were not prepared to parent another child. By contrast, the embryo placed has a different story: at the time of his conception, his parents deeply longed for a child or twins to parent. Because of medical and lab decisions, he was not included in the pair of embryos offered that opportunity. This knowledge could prompt an embryo-placed offspring to feel a profound sense of displacement. And since all of us sometimes wonder how we landed in our families, we imagine he may face a lifetime of recurring feelings that he is the wrong person in the wrong family. Knowing his genetic family may help answer some of his questions but could further intensify his sense of disconnection. We worry about how embryo-placed offspring will accept their families, and whether they will have feelings of anger, loss, confusion and resentment towards the medical caregivers and their birth parents.

The story of a child created through egg donation is fundamentally different from that of an embryo-placed offspring in several respects. First, in terms of genetic ties, the child created by egg donation does not have full siblings being raised by their genetic parents. In addition, this child has a genetic link to his/her father and to the father's entire family, past, present and future. And perhaps most significant for the child created through egg donation, there never were other intended parents. He has the opportunity to be raised by the people who sought to be his parents from the start.

DONOR FAMILY CONCERNS

Embryo placement raises questions not only for the offspring for whom an adoption was planned but also for the entire original family. Even recipient parents who do not plan to maintain contact with their child's donor family will recognize that the genetic family played—and continues to play—an important role in their child's life. How can embryo-recipient parents escape from the somber awareness that the genetic parents—people who believe that life begins with an embryo—have to live with a feeling of estrangement from their biological offspring. We wonder, also, what the siblings, who were transferred to their intended mom as embryos, will feel knowing that others were placed with other families.

Because of these issues and others, many selecting embryo placement will choose an open arrangement. While this arrangement may spare the offspring—both placed and raised by the genetic parents—some bewilderment, it does not necessarily make things easy for both sets of parents. How can placing parents really anticipate how they will feel in the future as they watch others raise children they desperately wanted and worked so very hard to create? What might happen if one or more of the genetic parents' children become ill or have a disability, while the placed-out children thrive? Or what of the reverse? Will the donors feel guilt and will the recipient parents feel they are being judged for the way they handle these challenges?

COMPARING TRADITIONAL BIRTH PARENTS
AND EMBRYO DONOR PARENTS

Adoption has taught us that birth parents do not forget the children they placed for adoption and that many go on in their lives with a profound sense of loss. Since all members of the adoption triad—adoptees, adoptive parents and birth parents— are, in many ways, connected for life, the losses experienced by birth parents touch the hearts and minds of adoptees and adoptive parents.

We wonder if the long-term impact of placing an embryo will be any less painful than it is in traditional adoption. Although embryo-placing parents do not experience saying goodbye to a real live baby, they are raising a child or children conceived at the same time as the embryo(s) they donated. What will it be like for these parents when they watch their child or children grow and know that there could be a third or a fourth child in the family? We expect that those who have open placements will wonder what it would be like if that child had been part of their family. And for those with closed placements, there will inevitably be feelings about the child who is out there in the world.

Traditional adoption is a solution to a problem: a child needs a home. Embryo placement grows out of a different problem: people have turned to science in an effort to become parents and the science has yielded more "offspring" than the parents feel prepared to raise. For those who believe that life begins with an embryo (otherwise, they would probably discard the embryo or donate to science rather than choose adoption), this may be profoundly troubling. "Did we violate the natural order of things?" they may wonder. "Was it wrong for us to pursue assisted reproduction when this was the outcome? Have our lives become a science fiction story?" they may ask.

It is too soon to know how this will all play out. Having experienced the pain of infertility, embryo donor parents may feel grateful to be able to help others become parents. They may go on in their lives feeling content that their efforts to build a family brought additional new lives into the world. Or they may be burdened with feelings of loss and confusion, wondering if what happened was really meant to be.

As we said at the start of this book, assisted reproduction, egg donation and, here, embryo placement highlight the blessings and the curses of the "meant to be."

RISKS

In a sense, embryo placement is a step closer to pregnancy than egg donation and might therefore seem to have fewer risks. After all, the embryo already exists and simply needs to be transferred to a womb. By contrast, egg donation requires several preliminary steps—medical and psychological screening of the donor, stimulation, egg retrieval and, finally, fertilization. Still, we caution people considering this option now to think about what it will mean for them and their children to be pioneers in this new and uncharted form of family building.

Meet Angie and Gino

"Because that's the way it is." Gino, a 35-year-old electrician, hears these words a lot these days. His wife, Angie, also 35 and pregnant for the first time through embryo placement, invokes them a lot. When her parents ask her to explain why she and Gino chose to become parents through embryo placement, she responds, "Because that's the way it is." When friends ask her how she will explain things to her child, she says, "Because that's the way it is." When she anticipates talking with a pediatrician about the fact that the donor couple—Gino's former colleagues—used a donor egg, Angie says, "I'll tell her 'that's the way it is.'"

That's the way it is. Angie and Gino, both first-generation Italian-Americans, never anticipated being trailblazers. When they set out to become parents five years ago, they assumed it would all happen the old-fashioned way. Indeed, Angie did conceive easily but that pregnancy ended in miscarriage. Another treatment ended in miscarriage, followed by a third pregnancy which proved ectopic. Along the way, the couple learned that Gino had serious defects in his sperm, that Angie's tubes were blocked and, while the physicians were at it, her eggs were "just so-so." The couple was exploring adoption when they received a call from Maria, an acquaintance. "I hear that the two of you are going through infertility. Remember Pat and Ryan? They went through infertility, had a little boy and decided not to have more children. They've been looking everywhere for a couple to adopt their frozen embryos. There are three of them."

"For a few seconds, I didn't know what to do. I had never really heard of embryo donation, let alone think of doing it ourselves. I assumed, once we heard that Gino's sperm was bad, that we'd use donor sperm. But when we tried it for one cycle, Gino became depressed. He said he'd feel left out if it worked. We were glad when it didn't."

Once Angie and Gino decided they needed to be "on equal footing with a child," they knew that neither egg donation nor donor sperm would work for them. Adoption was attractive but the costs were discouraging, especially for Angie and Gino who had full insurance coverage for all forms of treatment, including gamete donation and embryo placement. Then came Maria's call and it set a whole new process in motion.

Angie and Gino did not enter into embryo placement lightly. They talked a lot together and then talked with Pat and Ryan. The two couples agreed that they would be fully open about how their families were formed. The children would grow up knowing each other and would share important occasions. Both couples met with lawyers and with mental health counselors. Angie says that each step along the way confirmed to her that this was the right thing to do.

"I'm not an overly religious person, but I do have faith. I decided that God had things happen for a reason and then brought Pat and Ryan back into our lives for a reason. It feels like fate or destiny. And that's the way it is."

Sperm donation versus egg donation

Sounds like an odd choice, doesn't it, for a couple reading a book about egg donation because they need eggs to also consider using donated sperm? Since an egg and a sperm are both essential ingredients in pregnancy, why would anyone be choosing between them? In fact, there are two groups of couples who could find themselves in the position of choosing between donor eggs and donor sperm.

FAMILIES WITH GENETIC ISSUES

Couples in which both partners are carriers of a serious genetic condition have two options if they want to avoid transmitting that condition to their child: they can do IVF with PGD, something which is very complicated and expensive, or they can eliminate one of them as a carrier.

Take Alice and Larry, for example. Both are cystic fibrosis carriers and the parents of two sons, Matt and Alex. Matt has CF; Alex does not. Alice and Larry want another child but are afraid to roll the dice again. They can try IVF with PGD or they can decide to go with donor eggs or donor sperm. The obvious advantage of donor sperm is that it is much less costly and does not require assisted reproductive technology. However, with donor sperm, Larry is very much out of the pregnancy loop—Alice has both a genetic and a gestational tie to their next child and he has neither. If they choose egg donation, it will be more costly, but it will offer the couple parity—each will play a crucial role in bringing their child into this world.

UNEXPLAINED INFERTILITY

Although many people with unexplained infertility do learn more when they try IVF, there remain couples whose infertility continues to be entirely unexplained, even after IVF. They could try preimplantation genetic screening (PGS) or they can introduce either donated sperm or eggs to see if that makes a difference. Their decisions will be influenced by whether either or both partners have children and by costs, since donor sperm is much less expensive than egg donation.

Gestational care/surrogacy versus egg donation

In the early years after the development of IVF, when the procedure was experimental and not very successful, couples with female infertility problems had limited treatment options. Commercial surrogacy arrived to fill a gap. Those who wanted to have a biological connection to one parent sometimes turned to surrogacy as an alternative to adoption. With surrogacy, a woman willing to bear a child for another couple enters into a pre-conception adoption agreement with a couple. She agrees to become pregnant by being inseminated with the male partner's sperm and to place the child with the couple following birth in a legal process very akin to a step-parent adoption. This option was pursued by a number of infertile couples in the 1970s, but ceased to be widely sought once IVF was improved. For one thing, women who were unable to conceive because of blocked or absent fallopian tubes now had a greater chance to become pregnant. For another, IVF soon made egg donation possible, enabling a woman with a functioning uterus to carry and deliver her baby.

Finally, IVF made it possible for couples to create their own embryos and have them transferred to another woman if the intended mother was unable to gestate them. This woman became known as a gestational carrier and we will refer to the experience she undertakes as gestational care, although you may also hear it referred to as gestational surrogacy.

So what became of traditional surrogacy? It continues to have a place for some couples. They include couples in which the woman can neither produce viable eggs nor carry a pregnancy. Such couples can combine egg donation and gestational care, but may choose not to do so either for financial reasons and logistical reasons (surrogacy can be a very simple, low-tech process) or perhaps because a special person in their lives has volunteered to be their surrogate.

Surrogacy occasionally has a place for gay couples, and some prefer it to combining egg donation and gestational care, both because it is less costly and medically invasive and because they feel it will be less confusing for a child. However, many gay couples are reluctant to turn to traditional surrogacy. They worry that the surrogate, who is truly the child's birth mother, may change her mind and may then have parenting rights. Many also feel that they are looking for different qualities in an egg donor than in a surrogate and prefer to seek those qualities in two different women. Finally, they look at surrogacy through the child's lens and wonder how a child will comprehend that his birth mother entered into a pre-conception adoption arrangement.

Gestational carrier with egg donation

We turn now to an option that has become more common in recent years: gestational care with egg donation. This is often an option for gay male couples, but it is also one for heterosexual couples who have started down one path and then reached a second fork in the road. Namely, they have decided on egg donation only to find there is also a uterine issue or they have chosen a gestational carrier and now need an egg donor as well.

Meet Lee and Jim

I (Ellen) first met Lee and Jim three years ago. At the time, Lee, who was in her early 40s, was reeling from her infertility and the growing awareness that it was unlikely she would bear a child using her own eggs. She was angry, sad and confused. Then she and Jim took a trip to a beach resort. When she returned, something was different.

"I saw Anna at water's edge," Lee told me. Anna is the name that she and Jim had chosen for their first-born if they had a girl, and Lee was pretty certain she would have a girl. Then Dylan, her son, would come. Lee went on to tell me what it was like to see Anna as she stood on the sand. "Anna called to me. She said, 'Mommy, I'm coming.'" As she spoke, I could see that Lee was visibly relieved. She was actually happy. She said she knew now that Anna could come to her from a donor's eggs. "It will still be Anna. She will still be my baby."

I would like to say that Lee and Jim's journey to parenthood was easy from this point forth, but it was not. Lee and Jim set out to find a donor and, in short order, were delighted to locate someone who felt just right. She was in New York City and so Lee and Jim traveled there to meet her. The meeting went very well and Lee, in particular, left the meeting all the more certain that her donor would help her bring Anna into the world.

It was not to be. Infertility has a way of throwing curve balls and it surely had one for Lee and Jim: their donor, who had donated before, was turned down by their clinic because she failed her genetic screening.

Having known how much they liked their donor and how certain they were that she would bring them Anna, I assumed it would be very difficult for Lee and Jim to move on to another donor. What I underestimated was the strength of Anna's voice. She had assured her parents that she was coming and that assurance enabled them, I now realize in retrospect, (to paraphrase President Obama) to pick themselves up, dust themselves off and take the steps necessary to bring Anna home. That meant finding another donor, something they did remarkably quickly and with inspiring optimism.

"We've found her," Lee told me. And indeed they had. As wonderful as their first donor had been, Sandra was even better. They found her warmer, more engaging, more enthusiastic than their very lovely first donor. Once again, Lee and Jim were certain they had found "the one." This time things went well with her clinic screening and, before long, Sandra was officially Lee and Jim's donor. Her cycle went well: 12 eggs were retrieved and fertilized; six were frozen, two were transferred and one became Anna.

As she anticipated, Lee loved being pregnant. She loved the feeling of her baby growing inside her and, as the pregnancy unfolded, she became increasingly confident in the rightness of the choices she and Jim had made. All went well, and when Lee arrived at Brigham and Women's Hospital in Boston, at full term and in labor, she and Jim were filled with excitement, knowing that in a few hours Anna would be in their arms. What they didn't know was that within a few hours Lee would be in the intensive care unit fighting for her life and Jim would be holding baby Anna, facing a collision of emotions of overwhelming fear and a father's love.

Thankfully, Lee, who had suffered from a ruptured placenta, was in a superb hospital. The skilled care she received, combined with this loving mother's fierce will to live, pulled her through the crisis. Although she endured several days in the hospital and weeks at home recuperating, Lee was finally Anna's mom and the joy she felt surely eclipsed the physical pain and emotional trauma of her ordeal. Most important, it helped her cope with the entirely unexpected loss of her uterus and, with it, the ability to bring Dylan into the world with one of the cryopreserved embryos.

I saw Lee and Jim again last week. Lee came in with a big smile on her face and said, "This has been the best year of my life. I am so happy in so many, many ways." These words were not completely unexpected because I knew how much Lee had longed for Anna and how overjoyed she must be to finally welcome her home. However, I was also aware of what a difficult time Lee had had recovering from her emergency surgery and coping with more reproductive losses. Given all the challenges she faced, I was especially moved to hear and see Lee's joy.

"We're here to talk about a gestational carrier." Lee told me. "We have embryos and want to bring Dylan home."

"But what if it is another girl?" I asked.

"Dylan can be a girl's name as well as a boy's name," Lee smiled.

Adoption versus egg donation

Adoption, like egg donation, comes in various shapes and sizes. Domestic adoption, international adoption, same-race adoption, transracial adoption, infant adoption and older child adoption, the adoption of children who are healthy or of those who have various levels of health issues are all questions one must consider in making a decision to adopt.

The decision to choose adoption over egg donation or vice versa is ultimately, like most other important decisions in life, a matter of the heart. People can (and should) go to great lengths to analyze the pros and cons of their decision, but, ultimately, they are guided by what feels right. Nonetheless, if you are deciding between egg donation and adoption, you are likely to take the following into account.

IMPORTANCE OF PREGNANCY

If there is one single factor that clearly distinguishes the two paths to parenthood—especially for women—it is pregnancy. With egg donation, you have it; with adoption, you don't.

For some, pregnancy is an essential ingredient in a parent–child relationship. They feel that bonds between mother and child begin in utero and that a child benefits from hearing both of his parents' voices in the months before birth. They also value pregnancy because they know that what a woman eats and does not eat, drinks and does not drink during pregnancy can play a role in a newborn's health. In addition, some would-be parents look forward to pregnancy as a countdown to parenthood, anticipating nine months of preparation for a child's arrival.

Not everyone feels that pregnancy is important for them. If you have suffered devastating pregnancy losses, you may feel that pregnancy brings enormous pain and suffering. Or if you have had difficult pregnancies, marred by severe nausea, depression or physical illness, you may no longer feel that pregnancy is a perfect state. You may be among those who feel that pregnancy is a means to an end: parenthood.

Feelings about pregnancy often change in the course of infertility diagnosis and treatment. Some who initially had little interest in pregnancy find themselves longing for it. Others may find themselves moving in the reverse direction, seeing pregnancy as an experience that lasts nine months and parenthood as one that lasts a lifetime and is available without pregnancy.

The burgeoning field of epigentics has influenced how some intended parents think about egg donation and adoption. As *New York Times* medical writer Judith Shulevitz put it in her article "Why fathers really matter":

> Lately scientists have become obsessed with a means of inheritance that isn't genetic but isn't nongenetic either. It's epigenetic. "Epi" in Greek means "above" or "beyond." Think of epigenetics as the way our bodies modify their genetic makeup. Epigenetics describes how genes are turned on and off. (Shulevitz 2012)

Shulevitz goes on in her article to make a case for why what a father eats and drinks, thinks and feels, experiences and doesn't experience shapes his unborn child. Add this to the increasingly widespread acceptance of the role of epigenetics in pregnancy and we see more reasons why intended parents value and seek pregnancy.

RELATIONSHIP WITH THE CHILD
Everyone who sets out to be a parent wants to have a child they will love and cherish and who will feel authentically their child. For many, adoption feels like an incredible leap of faith. In signing

on to adopt, they feel they are making a lifelong commitment to a total stranger. This is daunting. A common concern voiced by prospective adoptive parents is, "I fear I will be living with a stranger."

Of course, some of this fear is based on a misunderstanding of how bonding and attachment works between human beings. Some assume that real bonding is a result of a nine-month gestation, and they wonder if they could ever attach to a child not genetically related to them. The truth is that bonding is an emotional connection between human beings that is based on a growing sense of the ability to trust one another. Those of us who will be parenting in pairs have already proven to ourselves that we can attach to someone genetically unrelated to us: we share an attachment with our partner.

Still, for some would-be parents, egg donation feels like less of an emotional stretch than adoption. They are reassured by the fact that the child will have a genetic connection to the father and, with intrafamily egg donation, to both parents. They are reassured, also, by the fact that the mother will have a gestational connection to the child. Although no one knows for sure what an unborn child feels and experiences, would-be parents often feel that it is important for their unborn child to know in utero that he is loved and eagerly awaited.

Others see bonding and attachment through a different lens. Some feel it will be much easier for the two of them to connect with a child that is adopted into the family with no genetic connection to either parent than it will would be to face what for them is the more complicated task of raising a child with a genetic connection to just one of them.

Egg donation is also attractive because it offers couples the opportunity to be present at the creation. Yes, the donor is an essential player, but the child conceived, is *intended to be your child*. Although you may have questions about whether a child conceived with donated gametes will have a difficult time understanding the donor's motivations, you may feel reassured that your child is unlikely to experience the feelings of rejection and loss that are so often troubling to adoptees.

HEALTH OF THE CHILD

Almost everyone wants a healthy child. Certainly, there are people who seek to adopt a child with a special need, but, for the most part, intended parents hope that the child who enters their family will be healthy, physically and emotionally. So what is the more likely way to have a healthy child—egg donation or adoption?

Some say adoption. When you adopt a newborn child, the child has been born and assessed by a hospital pediatrician who will be discharging a healthy baby to your care unless you voluntarily accept a child with a medical problem. Egg donation offers no such sureties. With egg donation, you have a pregnancy and you get what you get, just as you would in using your own eggs to conceive. A child born as a result of egg donation, like any other baby, can be born with any number of anomalies. (Between 1% and 4% of all babies are born with some genetic anomaly and there are some reports of this being slightly higher in IVF offspring.)

"On the other hand," would-be parents say, "we can pick the genes, do our best to 'control' the prenatal care, and we don't have to worry about our child being harmed by poor foster or institutional care."

Both views are accurate. With adoption, you get a healthy baby or toddler or young child, but you have little, if any, say in selecting his birth parents and you have no say in where he was before coming to you. Egg donation offers the father's genes on one side and the opportunity to select a donor—whether known or anonymous—for her genetic makeup. And it offers the intended parents the opportunity to control—as best anyone can—the prenatal environment and to make obstetrical choices.

FEELINGS OF FAMILY CONTINUITY

What does it mean to carry on a family line? In some families, any child who enters a family is a fully fledged member of the family tree, regardless of whether they were adopted or conceived with donor assistance. However, others view family continuity through a different lens. For them, it is difficult to "graft" someone onto the family tree.

For those who subscribe to the "any child of ours is part of the lineage of our family" perspective, it doesn't much matter whether they choose egg donation or adoption, at least as far as family continuity is concerned. However, those who regard genetic and/or gestational ties as very significant are likely to see egg donation as less of a stretch than adoption. Certainly, that will be the case on the father's side of the family, but perhaps also for the mother, since this child, although not her genetic offspring, was born to her.

Then comes the question of how important it is to feel a family tie to generations past and future. Although this is a compelling need for some, it is relatively unimportant for others. In the course of doing adoption home studies, I (Ellen) have met several couples who chose to adopt without ever trying to have a biological child. Some had something in their genetic heritage that they preferred not to pass on, but others did not. In both instances they seemed somewhat puzzled that people would feel a desire to carry on a bloodline.

EFFICACY

Will it work? Most people who are comparing egg donation and adoption have met with disappointments and frustrations along their path to parenthood. They want to find a light at the end of the tunnel and to head for it. How do egg donation and adoption compare?

Adoption is a sure bet. It will work. That doesn't mean that it will be easy or that it will necessarily work on the first try. Some would-be parents from non-traditional situations (age, sexual orientation, single status, etc.) may need to be more flexible when it comes to the age of the child and/or country of origin. Adoption can include fall-throughs when a new mother decides to parent her baby herself rather than go ahead with a planned adoption. Despite disappointments and frustrations along the way, those who persevere succeed in adopting.

Egg donation is not a sure bet. It has a good success rate, especially for those who are able to try more than once or twice. However, there are those who try egg donation and do not achieve successful pregnancies. When this occurs, some move on to adoption, having lost time and money along the way. Lost time may not be of particular concern for younger couples, but for those who first try egg donation in their mid to late 40s, the delay in time may significantly reduce their adoption options.

For couples who hope to have more than one child, egg donation offers a potential bonus: twins. Although many egg donation pregnancies are singletons, twins come along often, especially if two or more embryos are transferred. The arrival of twins, while challenging physically and in other ways, may provide parents with the instant family they longed for. Fertility centers, recognizing the increased risks associated with multiples, remind patients that it is important to transfer as few embryos as possible in order to minimize the chance of multiples. Unfortunately, many couples have struggled so long and want children so desperately that it is hard not to think "the more the merrier"—not "the more the scarier"—when warned of multiples.

FINANCIAL COSTS

Both egg donation and adoption involve substantial costs, and, with each option, there is a range of costs which vary depending on where you live. In the US, domestic infant adoption currently costs between $25,000 and $50,000. Adoption of older and special needs children through state social service agencies in the US can involve very few, if any, out-of-pocket expenses. The US Government provides families with $13,360 towards their adoptions in the form of a tax credit (this is the 2011 figure—it changes yearly and is phased out over a certain income level). In addition, many US employers, including major companies, universities and medical institutions, offer employees an adoption benefit, often in the $5000–10,000 range.

Egg donation costs vary worldwide and costs per cycle can be a good deal lower than adoption. If a successful pregnancy is achieved on a first or second cycle, the costs of egg donation may well be lower than adoption. However, if egg donation does not work and a couple moves on to adoption—or to trying with other donors—costs mount.

ETHICAL CONSIDERATIONS

Dr. Aaron Lazare, the Celia and Isaac Haidak Professor in Medical Education at the University of Massachusetts Medical School and founder of the Center for Adoption Research, said the following of adoption: "What other institution is socially correct, morally correct, politically correct, economically correct?" Indeed, adoption, which finds homes for children who need them, is "ethically correct." Yes, there have been black market adoptions and other deplorable practices, but here, at the start of the twenty-first century, adoption is governed by state, national and, with the passing of the Hague Convention, international regulations. These laws strive to eliminate any risk of "baby selling," or of birth parents or entrepreneurs profiting in other ways from adoption.

In the United States, egg donation is essentially an unregulated industry. The American Society for Reproductive Medicine offers guidelines for practice, but there are no enforceable rules and regulations. At this point in time, virtually anyone can call themselves an egg donor agency and recruit young women as donors. Similarly, nearly everyone can present at a medical clinic and pretty much demand medical assistance with egg donation. No laws or guidelines exist to say this woman should not donate her eggs or that couple should not be permitted to create a child through egg donation.

In the absence of regulations, egg donor programs and fertility clinics are left to regulate themselves. This is extraordinarily difficult, since even those who feel strongly about working in what they see as an ethically sound way are met with challenges.

Another concern raised by egg donation is whether it is ethically correct to intentionally create a child who will not be raised by both of his biological parents. Some say, "Of course, the child will be created in love and will be deeply wanted." However, others will argue that donor offspring enter life facing an avoidable loss—the loss of a genetic connection to one's parents.

HUMANITARIAN CONSIDERATIONS
No one should ever feel that a history of infertility instructs them to be humanitarians. However, for some, the opportunity to do good, to make a difference in a child's life, to offer a home to someone who would otherwise not have one is inviting. We spoke before about the "blessing and the curse of the meant to be" and adopting a child often feels as if things "happen for a reason."

LEGAL CONSIDERATIONS
When people have struggled long and hard to bring a child into their families, the last thing they want is to fear losing that child. While neither adoption nor egg donation nor anything else can fully protect people from accidents, illness and other tragic losses, there are legal safeguards that protect adoptive and egg donation parents from loss due to others claiming parental rights.

Egg donation works fairly simply. A legal contract is generally signed at the time eggs are donated. This contract clearly establishes the fact that the donor does not have and will never have parental rights. For an expanded discussion of this, see Chapter 5.

Adoption is more complicated legally. In nearly every state in the US, there is a window of time. Most often a matter of days, (occasionally a matter of weeks or months) during which a woman can change her mind about whether to place her child. Good adoption professionals educate would-be parents about these waiver periods when a placement is at legal risk and may even suggest that the child go to foster care during that window of opportunity. Depending upon the state and the country a child is born in, an adoption may be more or less legally secure. When the participants live in more than one state, the laws of both states must be followed. International adoption involves the laws of more than one state/country. Working with professionals who are knowledgeable about the laws and are committed to following them ethically is the most important guarantee that a finalized adoption is completely safe. What is important for people to know when they are deciding between egg donation and adoption is that there are many adoptions that are entirely secure from the time of placement. These include adoptions in countries where the adoption is finalized in the country within days of the child being placed with his family and in US states that have no revocation period, meaning that if a child's birth parents surrender their parental rights according to predetermined state protocol, they cannot change their minds and return seeking custody of the child.

SOCIAL NORMS

Adoption has existed throughout history and has long been accepted as a means of family building. Egg donation arrived only in the 1980s and is therefore less familiar to most people. For some, egg donation still feels weird, unnatural, "like science fiction." People who react this way and who are comfortable with adoption are likely to choose the path that is familiar.

Some are drawn to egg donation because it is invisible. With adoption—especially transracial adoption—everyone knows. For those who want to be sure they fit in and look like everyone else, egg donation is attractive. Many feel that their child is the only one who really needs to know how their family was built.

TALKING WITH CHILDREN ABOUT THEIR ORIGINS

Although we like to think that everyone who adopts a child or has one through egg donation will feel comfortable and confident talking with their child about how they entered the family, some intended parents are understandably uneasy. Thankfully, their discomfort tends to diminish once there are real, live children in their homes, but, in advance, the anxiety can be daunting. "How will we talk with our child without upsetting him and feeling rejected ourselves?"

In thinking about talking with children, some prefer the simplicity of an adoption story to the newfangled egg donation tale. Yes, adoption involves loss and possibly feelings of rejection, but it feels simple and uncomplicated because adoption is familiar, public, widely accepted and respected. Parents can talk with their children, confident that the children will know others who joined their families through adoption. In addition, in recent years adoption has become very fashionable, so much so that there are adoption specials on TV, feature stories of celebrity adoptions and so on.

For an expanded discussion about talking with children, please see Chapter 8. However, we want to take a moment here to remind readers that although egg donation is newer and provides fewer models to follow, families can learn from both adoption and from donor sperm offspring, and they can have wonderful conversations within the privacy of their own homes. Remember that children are very self-centered and love to hear stories about themselves. Instead of approaching disclosure from a self-conscious "What will I do wrong?" perspective, we encourage parents to think about the positive conversations they can look forward to having with their children. How wonderful it can be to tell a child how much he was wanted, how thrilled you were to know he was coming, how much joy he brought when he finally arrived.

Sadly, some considering egg donation don't see it this way. When they think about talking with their future children, they are filled with a kind of irrational fear and anxiety. Some comfort themselves by saying, "We don't really have to tell if we decide not to." Others acknowledge the need to tell, but anticipate that, when the time comes, they will want to avoid or postpone conversations. Again, we remind readers that this is a happy story. Telling it proudly and confidently and with joy will help provide your child with important foundations of self-esteem and belonging: "We wanted you, someone helped us make you, we loved seeing you grow in Mommy's tummy and we were over the top with happiness when you were born." (The donor doesn't see the egg as a potential child—she sees it as an ingredient to help another family create a child.) The adoption story includes some of this joy, but there is also the other side of things—there were other potential parents and, for whatever reason, they were unable to parent at that time.

Existing family composition

Parents look at the family they already have when it comes time to consider egg donation or adoption. Some who have a biological child choose egg donation hoping for another pregnancy and a child who will be half genetically connected to his sibling. They may look at egg donation and observe how similar it is to regular biological parenting—the couple plans for the child, the mother carries the baby, the dad is the genetic father and the couple gets to share pregnancy, labor and delivery. It all seems remarkably familiar.

Others see things through another lens. Adoption offers an opportunity to expand the family in a different way. Parents always worry about comparing their children and about whether having a second child will live up to their experience with a first. Adoption—especially transcultural or transracial adoption— invites parents to depart from comparisons and to celebrate differences.

Since more and more people are marrying for a second time after divorce or the death of a spouse, there are many couples considering egg donation or adoption when they are older and when one or both has other children. These experiences will also influence their decision. When a man who has never had a child marries a woman who is the biological mother of her child(ren), egg donation can be especially attractive. When both partners have had children, adoption offers them the opportunity to share a new experience together.

Your child's story

Everyone has a personal narrative about how they entered their family. "I was planned," "I was named after my grandfather," "I was an accident," "My parents were still trying for a girl" and so on. Joining one's family through adoption or egg donation surely adds a dimension to the story. We think it safe to say that egg donation is never a first choice and that adoption is usually not a first choice. One of the reasons why it is so important for parents to really come to terms with the second choices they make along the way is that we don't want to have children whose personal narrative includes "second choice."

Loving parents will do what they can to convey to their children that they were very much wanted and are deeply loved, regardless of how the parents originally felt about a second-choice path to parenthood. For some parents, this is easier to do with adoption: they feel that the child can develop a positive personal narrative based on the story that he was born to parents who loved him but could not parent him, and that his "now and forever" parents were thrilled to have him. For these parents, egg donation provides more challenges. They wonder how a child forms a secure personal narrative based on the knowledge that he came from two women.

Others disagree. "How hard is it," they ask, "for a child to see one woman as offering important baby-making ingredients to two eager parents in need of them?" What a happy, positive personal story these children will form, one built on the solid foundation of knowing their parents intentionally created them to be part of the family they live with and belong in.

THE FAMILY STORY

Finally, we come to your family story. Anyone who considers egg donation and most people who consider adoption have to relinquish their original vision of what their family would look like. Indeed, most parents are forced to abandon this fantasy somewhere in their lives, although, for many, it comes when they are raising children, not bringing them into the family.

So what, then, does your second-choice family story look like? Again, how you look at this may be determined by whether you have children already and whether this is a first marriage for each of you. For some, egg donation feels like less of a second choice because it feels "closer to what we originally wanted"—to be pregnant, to share childbirth, to have at least some genetic connection.

Faced with loss and disappointment, others take a different approach to creating a second-choice family story. "If it has to be a different family from the one we imagined, then let it really look and feel and be a different family." Some who choose adoption, especially an international and/or transracial adoption, discover that family building can truly be an unexpected adventure, filled with travel and cultural rewards they never anticipated.

Again, we remind you that whether you choose adoption or egg donation, it is *your* family story. Write it with thought and with pride. With adoption, you will encounter a story that has already begun but which you can build upon wisely. With egg donation, you have the opportunity to write the story from the start. Make it a story you will feel proud to share with your child.

Meet Terry and Mark

Terry and Mark were "on the fence" for a long time. When they married, at 45 and 35, both knew it was unlikely that Terry would be able to become pregnant with her own eggs. Since she had been thinking about adopting as a single woman for several years, Terry simply assumed that Mark would be happy to join her in an adoption. Mark has a cousin who recently adopted from China and, perhaps more to the point, Mark joined his own family through adoption. And so it came as a surprise to Terry when Mark said, "I'd rather do egg donation."

There they were—Terry preferred adoption and Mark preferred egg donation. Each voiced very compelling reasons for their choice. For Terry, pregnancy at 45 or 46 seemed scary and, she felt, "unnatural." She described egg donation as "sci-fi" and embraced adoption as "a good thing for everyone concerned." She pointed to Mark and his family as "great proof that adoption works" and wondered why people would want to create a child through eggs donated from a stranger. In addition, she reminded Mark that his birth sister is schizophrenic and questioned whether they should be worried about "passing on mental illness genes."

Mark, by contrast, advocated for egg donation. He spoke poignantly to Terry of his desire to have a biological offspring and also of his wish to share a pregnancy with her. He spoke with some skepticism about adoption "these days," contrasting current practice with the good matching that he felt went on at the time his parents adopted. However, he added that he would be willing to adopt if they had a child through egg donation first or if they tried egg donor and it didn't work.

This was not an easy situation. Terry and Mark had each waited a long time to find the right life partner and both agreed they were lucky to have found each other. But how were they to resolve what felt like an impasse? Many discussions ensued, including several with a counselor, who helped them to listen carefully to the other's concerns and desires. Ultimately, it was Terry who decided she could make a shift in her thinking. These were Terry's words: "I grew up knowing my biological family so I can't say, first hand, what it feels like to not know people to whom you are connected genetically. Yes, Mark was lucky enough to find his birth family as an adult, but when I thought about it, I realized that did not erase the impact of the years of not knowing. When I thought about it that way, I decided that Mark deserved to enjoy a parent–child relationship that included a genetic connection, not only because it was important for him as a father, but also because he felt so strongly about it for his child."

Not being parents or, in the case of secondary infertility, being a one-child family

There are individuals and couples who travel a long, arduous road through infertility and, after examining many options, decide not to pursue parenthood through adoption or any of the third-party collaborative options. Some of you already have a child or children and decide to stay with the family you have rather than try to add to it via an alternative route. Others do not have children but realize that alternative paths to parenthood are not right for them.

There are couples who start down the road of infertility diagnosis, who travel a long way through treatment or who carefully examine alternative paths to parenthood and ultimately conclude that their lives are full and satisfying without children. Many are couples who met later in life and who rushed into infertility treatment because they knew that time was running out. Some find, as they look at their options, that their glass is mostly full. They may be approaching mid-life and conclude that there are other satisfying ways to spend their time. For some who have begun to feel this way, it may come as a big relief to step back, celebrate the relationship you have and enjoy some of the fruits of your labors. Parenthood can be satisfying, gratifying and pleasurable, but it is also frustrating, stressful and, sadly, for some, it brings sorrow.

If you already have a child, you may conclude that remaining with one child is your best option. There was once a stigma about only children, but, thankfully, that stigma has vanished. Today, people are creating all kinds of families, making one-child families more common and less isolated. If you have a healthy child, who is thriving, you may feel it is time to count blessings rather than seek new ones.

Full circle—coming back to the option of using donated eggs

If you have taken the time—most likely days or weeks or, in some cases, even months—to consider carefully the options we've mentioned above (other collaborative reproductive options, adoption, accepting your life as full just as it is), if your infertility issues make you a candidate to try using egg donation and if you just don't feel ready to make any of those leaps, you've come full circle from the beginning of this chapter. Egg donation remains an option you need and want to explore more fully.

We may be leaving some of our readers here. There are those of you who will decide not to pursue egg donation, perhaps because of something we have said in this chapter or in a previous one. But many of you will move on. We hope the chapters that follow will provide you with practical information and emotional support as you pursue egg donation.

– 4 –

Choosing Your Donor

Here you are at another fork in the road. You've explored other options and have decided to move forward with egg donation. One big decision has been made, but another sits before you: identifying your donor. For a few of you, the decision may seem straightforward: you have a sister, cousin or friend who has offered to donate to you and you are delighted by her offer. However, for most people, deciding on the type of donor they desire and then finding that specific donor are formidable decisions.

In this chapter we will look at how people identify their donors. In keeping with the central themes of this book, we encourage you to look at each of your options through the bifocal lens of the best interests of the child and of parental satisfaction and security. Which egg donor choice can you look back on ten years from now and be able to say, "She was absolutely the right choice"? "By choosing her we were able to have a child whom we love and cherish and with whom we can speak openly and proudly about the way he joined our family. We feel grateful to our donor, who gave us a gift that enriched our lives and those of our families now and for future generations. We believe that, by giving to us, the donor enriched her own life as well as ours."

As we introduce some of the ways people choose donors, we acknowledge that our readership is international and that some of you may be subject to specific government regulations that limit or define your choices in a donor.

What type of donor is best for you?

There are four general categories of egg donors:

1. Family members—including sisters, cousins and, in some instances, nieces.

2. Friends and acquaintances—including close friends and casual acquaintances.

3. Program-recruited donors—including women who receive financial compensation to provide eggs either anonymously or on an open basis.

4. Women who donate to egg banks—these are women who are not donating to a specific individual or couple but rather contributing their eggs to an egg bank where they are cryopreserved for future use.

As you face the decision of what type of donor is right for you, we encourage you to step back and consider what you are looking for in a donor. Although every individual and couple have different qualities they value in a donor, the following are what we have found to be the most common priorities.

Fertility

Everyone wants a fertile donor. After all, why would you seek her eggs if these eggs are unlikely to result in a successful pregnancy? As you think of the four categories of donors from the standpoint of fertility, you will be taking into account the donor's age, whether she has had children and, if so, how recently, and, in some instances, whether she has donated before and, if so, whether it resulted in a successful pregnancy.

The child's story and best interests of children

Although, as recipients, you may have different preferences and priorities, we would venture to say that *all of you* ultimately have the *same* goal: to have a child who thrives in your family.

Central to your child's well-being will be his comfort with the story of how he joined your family. Unlike adoptive parents, who come into their child's life when the story has already been partially written, with egg donation you *create* the story. Your choice of donor and how you collaborate with her in the process will be crucial building blocks for that story.

Appearance

As you look for a donor, appearance is likely to be part of your decision making. Unlike other traits, such as interests, talents, intelligence, which are shaped in large measure by environment, physical traits such as height, skin color, eye and nose shape are part of the mixture of inherited characteristics. We have found that most recipients are not looking for a donor who looks just like the intended mom, but you are likely to seek someone who resembles you in some important ways. As one recipient said, "I'm very tall and that is the first thing people notice about me. I chose a tall donor because I wanted to do what I could to ensure height." Another recipient, who found her donor at a program, said, "I approached it with the 'second cousin test.' I'd look at the women's photos and ask myself, 'Could this person be my second cousin?' Of course, I wasn't about to turn someone down who looked close enough to be a sister, but second cousin was good enough."

Health

Everyone seeking egg donation hopes to have a healthy child. Although there are countless physical and mental conditions that can be neither predicted nor avoided, the major mental illnesses and some physical illnesses have genetic components. Sorting through medical history and through your own reactions to particular conditions is difficult for most recipients. Many voice feelings of responsibility to the child, saying it is unfair to bring a medical problem into the family. However, when asked if they took family medical and mental health histories from people they dated, most intended parents laugh at the notion of vetting a prospective spouse for "good genes."

If you would have happily married someone whose family medical or mental health history includes some worrisome conditions, then why reject a donor with the same conditions? It seems that the difference has to do with intentionality. When people marry someone who may be passing something on to a child, they don't typically think, "I'm doing this to my child." However, in choosing a donor, we have found that many recipients do feel a responsibility to their child to screen out the "bad genes."

And what is a "bad gene"? We encourage you to distinguish between something that is common and not thought to have a strong genetic component and something that is deadly and transmitted almost always through genes. You may want to turn to your primary care doctor for advice in sorting this out. Remember also that your reproductive endocrinologist and your medical program's psychologist or social worker will weigh in on your donor's medical and mental health history and possibly recommend working with her.

Ethnicity

For some of us, our ethnic, religious and cultural histories are of primarily importance: they are central to who we are and we feel very strongly about passing them on to our children. While some of us feel these ethnic heritages can be passed on through environment and look forward to transmitting our heritage through its foods, customs and holidays, others feel that ethnicity is in the genes. If you find yourself in that camp, having a child who shares your ethnic heritage may be of paramount importance. I (Ellen) remember one American woman of Irish heritage whose husband is Jewish. She agreed to raise their children Jewish and so, when it came to finding a donor, she felt strongly that she wanted a full Irish donor: "I need to know I am passing on my heritage."

Character, personality and intelligence

Although the process of choosing a donor usually begins with focus on fertility and appearance, we have found that, as the process unfolds, character and personality play increasingly important roles in your decision making. Most everyone we meet wants a donor that they believe to be a "good" person. Many look for the following traits in a donor: kindness, compassion, optimism, self-confidence, goal orientation, strong family values, loyalty, altruism. Although these qualities may not be genetically transmitted, recipients want to feel confident that their child "comes from a good place."

Intelligence is also often a consideration in selecting a donor. Most recipients don't seem to be looking for a donor who is an academic superstar, but they want some evidence that she is a capable person, someone who can set goals for herself and achieve them.

Cost

While we hope you don't have to make your decisions solely on the basis of cost, we know that, for many of you considering egg donation, cost is a major factor.

Depending upon your financial situation, the fees to an agency, a lawyer and medical treatment may be of more or less concern. However, fees paid to the donor are of concern to all intended parents, regardless of financial resources. No one wants to raise a child who feels like a commodity. At the time of writing, there are several countries, including Germany, Norway, Austria and Canada, that ban any payment for egg donors and some, such as the UK, that cover reimbursement for time and effort. Children are unlikely to feel like the products of a sale when there is no payment to the donor. But what of the programs in the US that offer significant amounts of money to donors? What is a reasonable fee for her efforts and when is a fee "too high"?

In the United States (at the time of writing), fees above $8000–$10,000 are considered excessive. There are some programs that set a fee in the range of $5000–$7000 and offer it to all their donors. The idea of having a "one fee fits all" for donors makes sense to us as it affirms the concept that someone is being paid for time and effort, rather than being rewarded for high SATs, physical beauty or the fact that she produced 20 eggs last cycle. However, "one fee fits all" is rarely the case and, in practice, many programs offer donors more compensation when they have had successful donations in the past or because they have other physical or intellectual features that make them more desirable.

Ethical considerations

As much as you want to become pregnant and to experience the joy of welcoming a new baby into your family, you will want to feel confident that the decision to donate is right for your donor. As you think about which kind of donor to choose, you will want to confirm that she is someone who is making a decision with informed consent, free and clear of outside pressures or influences. You will want to feel that she will look back on the experience and feel it was the right decision. This is one of the reasons we raise concerns about high fees: they increase the risk that women will go through egg donation "for the money."

Our family

Your existing family composition will play some role in determining whom you select as your donor. Your race and whether you have children together or separately from earlier marriages will impact your decision making.

We will focus now on each kind of donor and look at her through the lens of the priorities we listed earlier: fertility; the child's story; appearance; health; ethnicity; character, personality and intelligence; cost; ethical considerations; and our family.

Intrafamily donation

For a number of reasons, intrafamily egg donation makes a lot of sense. It offers recipients the opportunity to parent a child with genetic connections to both of his parents. It provides the child with a positive message about how family members love, care and help each other. It avoids ethical concerns about payment for eggs since family members are rarely compensated. And it is more affordable because there will be no fees to agencies.

If only it were that simple. Most people seeking egg donation do not have a sister or other close family member who is ready, willing and able to donate. Some don't have a sister and those who do may find that she is not willing or she may not be able or she may be willing and able but not ready. For lots of reasons, most people seeking a donor have to look outside their families. Nonetheless, there are some recipients with family members who have offered to donate or whom they are considering asking. If you are among them, these are some of the things you will be thinking about regarding your donor.

Fertility

If you have a family member in mind, the first thing you need to clarify is whether your medical program will consider her to be a suitable candidate. Most often, intrafamily donations are limited to sister-to-sister and cousin-to-cousin donations, with donations from daughter to mother challenged for ethical reasons. Occasionally, there will be a niece-to-aunt donation. From a medical perspective, physicians will be looking for family members who are under 35 and who have had children, although most physicians will not turn away a sister who is over 35 and has not had a child.

What you are unlikely to know with your family member is how she will respond to the fertility medications. Unlike program-recruited donors, where there is often a history provided of her past cycles, or with egg bank donors, where the eggs are already retrieved and frozen, with a family member you will be basing fertility predictions solely on her lab results, her age and reproductive history.

The child's story

If there is a compelling reason to have a family member as your donor, it is for the child's story. How nice it could be to teach a child, from an early age, about love, loyalty and generosity within families—about what family members will do for each other and how much this means to the giver and the receiver.

In addition to the messages conveyed to a child about family bonds, intrafamily donation is an extension, in some ways, of practices that have existed throughout history. Dating back to biblical days, sisters have raised their sisters' children, grandparents have stepped in when the children of their children needed parenting. In many cultures, children belong to an extended family and grow up feeling close ties to people beyond their nuclear family.

So there are some substantial advantages to intrafamily donation, but it is not right for everyone. Some people feel that it would be confusing to the child, who would not be able to distinguish siblings from cousins, an aunt from a mom. If either the donor or the prospective recipient feels this way, intrafamily donation is not right for them.

Appearance

Will your family member pass "the second cousin test"? Probably, but not necessarily. Although one of the benefits of having a family member as donor is that you may share some physical resemblances, this is not always the case. There are families in which sisters look very different from each other and this is all the more likely with cousins. One recipient said, "I have two sisters and we all look completely different. I have dark hair, dark eyes and complexion, and one sister has blond hair and is fair. The third, believe it or not, is a redhead. I'd be happy having either of my sisters donate because we've already seen in our family that genes don't determine looks." Another recipient might feel very different about this, concerned that if she has a child that looks "just like my sister," the strong resemblance will draw constant attention to how the child was conceived.

Health

We spoke earlier about how people feel a responsibility to their children not to bring in genes that are not already in the family. But what if they are already there? What do you do if there are some family genes that you are not sure you want to pass on? Granted you would have taken that chance had you conceived on your own, but bringing in a family member as donor shifts things from the *assumption* that the genes could be passed on to making it a matter of choice. And to complicate things further, what if the identified family member has a condition that you do not have?

When you are thinking about a family member as donor, you will probably also be thinking a lot about her medical and mental health and how the donation might impact her. While you wouldn't want any harm to come to a donor you found in a program, with a sister or cousin you are probably paying much closer attention to the potential medical consequences of donation. Although there is no clear evidence that undergoing stimulation and/or retrieval increases a woman's risk of future infertility or of ovarian cancer, this is something on many people's minds. Frequently, recipients thinking about having a sister donate say, "I'm worried. What if something happens and she is unable to have children? What if years from now she develops ovarian cancer? Will we—or will she—look back and blame the treatment?"

Ethnicity

Family members share ethnic history, either in its entirety with sisters or partially with half-sisters and cousins, who could have a parent with a different ethnicity. This shared cultural history is so important to many recipients who feel comforted to know "My child is *really* Italian" or "This enables me to pass on my Portuguese heritage that is so central to who I am."

Character, personality and intelligence

We can pick our friends but not our family members. Some of us adore our sisters or cousins, and others of us experience them as difficult, competitive, stubborn and the like. If you are considering a family member as donor, it's probably important that you feel good about your donor's character and personality. While one might argue that these qualities may not be genetic and may not matter so much if your donor is a stranger, they surely matter if your donor is a family member. You will be seeing your donor and interacting with her for years to come. You don't want to have someone who will hold what she did for you over your head, reminding you that you owe her or you should be eternally grateful. In other words, while we observed earlier that most recipients seek a donor who they find to have good character and appealing personality, these traits are all the more important in a family member.

Intelligence is thought to be genetic, at least in part, and we have all learned that there are many forms of intelligence. Some of the brightest people you know may not be the ones who score highest on standardized tests or get great grades in school. One advantage to a family member is that you have a broader perspective on her intelligence. You've seen the way she lives her life, the choices she makes, the things she accomplishes, and you can feel comfortable—or not—with her level of intelligence.

Cost

Among the many benefits of a family member as donor is cost. With a family member, you will have legal costs and counseling costs and, depending on your insurance coverage, you may have medical costs, but you will save donor agency fees and you will most likely not be paying your family member a fee. That said, most recipients do feel strongly about giving their family member a substantial gift for donating. If your donor has children, a gift that many people are comfortable with is a donation to the children's college fund. If the donor does not have a family, sometimes the gift is shares in a mutual fund or a bond. Either way, the sentiment is usually the same: you are helping us build our future and we are similarly investing in your future. So the primary cost savings with family members as donors comes in agency fees.

Ethical considerations

Having a family member donate eliminates the ethical dilemmas that arise with donors who may be enticed by money. We're assuming that even if you are giving your intrafamily donor a substantial gift, she is not doing this for the money. However, with family members, other ethical issues arise, also related to her motivation for donating. Does she really want to give some of her eggs to you or is she doing this because she feels some pressure—whether overt or covert—to do so? If you are a cancer survivor or lost your ovaries in an accident, does your family member feel somehow obliged to do this for you? Other ethical issues arise if she has conflicts with her husband or partner about donating. What if she really wants to help you but faces objections from her partner? As with matters of character and personality, we have found that, in considering a family member as donor, recipients often raise the bar when it comes to confirming the ethical "rightness" of a donation.

Our family

The composition of your existing family will also influence how you think about intrafamily donation. If this is a second marriage and your husband has genetically related children and you do not, you may welcome intrafamily donation as a means of making a genetic contribution from "your side." If you and your husband have had a child together and face secondary infertility, a family member as donor may offer the closest thing to having another full biological child.

"Our family" can mean extended as well as nuclear family. Will you feel more—or less—comfortable in your extended family having an intrafamily donation. While this may seem like the most natural thing in the world in some families, there are others that might treat it as fuel for constant and unwelcome conversation.

Special considerations

If you are thinking of intrafamily donation, here are some special considerations unique to intrafamily donation.

WHAT IF YOUR PROSPECTIVE DONOR HAS NOT OFFERED?

You may have a family member who you think would be quite willing to donate but she has not offered. What do you do in this instance? How can you ask her to donate and how can you be prepared for her to say no? These are both huge challenges for many recipients for which we offer the following guidance.

If you are thinking about asking a family member to donate, you need to be absolutely certain you will be okay if she says no. You cannot ask her to do this if you anticipate you will be angry, hurt or resentful if she refuses. We realize that this is a tall order since this means so very much to you, and it must be hard to imagine that someone who loves you could turn you down for something that matters so much. "After all," you think, "if the tables were turned, I would surely do this for her." This doesn't matter. People are different and your sister or cousin may love you very much, want to help but still feel unable to donate. We encourage you to see it this way: if she says no, she is "unable," not "unwilling."

So how do you ask her in a way that gives her real permission to say no and that is not embarrassing or awkward for both of you? Our thought is that a letter is easier than a phone or in-person conversation. In a letter, you can carefully choose and craft your words and she has the chance to read and re-read them. A letter gives you the chance to say exactly what you want to say, without risk that you will fumble and put your foot in your mouth, and it gives her a chance to react in private. If you feel awkward sending her a letter, you can let her know there is something you want to discuss with her and you want to first introduce it in a letter.

What if you have more than one sister, more than one prospective donor?

For some recipients, there is only one family member who is a potential donor, but others have more than one prospect. What do you do if you have two or more people who might be willing to donate? You are likely to prefer one over the other, but that may not be so clear-cut. Perhaps you would choose one sister for her appearance and personality and the other for her age and fertility history. What you don't want to happen is to have one person left out or feeling that she was your back-up or second choice.

You have a few options. You can approach people one at a time, beginning with your "best" option, or you can write a group letter explaining what is going on, how you would be happy to have one of X number of family members donate and how decisions have to be made on the basis of health, fertility and so on. You can cast this larger net and see how people react. One advantage to this approach is that it makes it easier for any one donor to say no—she is less likely to feel put on the spot.

Should you find that you have more than one sister willing and able to donate to you, you will probably want to find ways to include the non-donating sister into your cycle, finding some role for her. As one recipient said, "We are three sisters who have been best friends all our lives. Now I will have a special bond with the sister who is donating, but I don't want our other sister to feel in any way 'out of the loop.' I want to find ways for her to feel that this is 'our family expanding project.'"

Friend or acquaintance donation

As we noted earlier, most of us have more friends than family members and more acquaintances than friends. In addition, we can have friends ten or more years younger than us. Hence, the potential field of donors is larger with friends and acquaintances than it is with family members. That said, many intended parents do a mental survey of the people they know and rapidly conclude they know no one whom they can ask or no one who will be a suitable donor. We are grateful to Kris Probasco, a social worker in Missouri and Kansas, for sharing with us her experiences helping people find known donors. Probasco says, "Over 75 percent of my practice is known donors. I help people network, encouraging them to tell everyone they know and ask them to tell everyone they know. Donors come forward. There are many instances where it really feels it was 'meant to be.'" Here are some things people consider in seeking a known donor.

Fertility

With friends and acquaintances, as with family members, you will be paying attention to her age and her reproductive history. Does she have children? If so, how old are they and did she have difficulty conceiving? Before you begin speaking with your prospective known donor, ask your physician what he or she recommends in terms of basic tests, such as FSH or AMH. You will want to do as much as you can to confirm her probable fertility early in the process so that you don't begin a series of important and deeply personal conversations only to be later met with disappointment.

The child's story

Friend-to-friend donation can offer a child a wonderful story about friendship. Acquaintance-to-acquaintance donation can offer a child a different kind of positive message: that we live in a world where people are willing to help others. Kris Probasco recommends that families planning known donation regard it as a friendship between two families who will remain in regular contact and see each other a few times a year. Most parents want to raise children who value friendship, who seek to do good deeds, who see themselves as part of a community and value acts and actions that serve to better the community. If you are thinking about having a friend or acquaintance donate, you may also welcome a story that you feel will make sense to your child. You will not be saying, "We're so lucky donor 458 helped us," but, rather, "Alison is so special to us. She was my friend in college and then she did the most wonderful thing—she helped us have you" or, "We were so lucky to have found Amelia, our friend Andrea's sister. Amelia heard about how much we wanted to be parents and said that she wanted to help us make that happen. Now she and her family have become our special friends."

Appearance

Your friend/acquaintance may look something like you or she may not. We have found that appearance often matters less to people when they know their donor and she is someone they like and feel close to. Sometimes the offer from a friend or co-worker is so unexpected, so sincere, so deeply appreciated, that you find you are more touched by who she is and what she wants to do than by how she looks. Or you may feel otherwise—touched and appreciative of her offer but reluctant to accept it because the child would simply look too different.

Health

An advantage to having a friend donate is that your child is more likely to have access to up-to-date family medical information throughout his life. In addition, you may feel more confident about the accuracy of the information than you would if reviewing a questionnaire from a donor agency. But, as with all donors, that question of "What are we bringing into the family?" is likely to arise with a friend. You know her and you know her family members, and you may find yourself sizing them up in terms of medical and mental health history. Again, we encourage you to distinguish between conditions that are common and not necessarily genetic and those that are devastating and have a strong genetic component.

Ethnicity

Your friend may be from your ethnic group or have a different heritage, and you will have to sort out, as with any non-family donor, how much shared ethnicity matters. For some of you, shared ethnicity will trump other factors and you might turn down a friend in favor of finding someone at an agency who shares your heritage. Or you may feel that some things matter less when you know the person involved and you are entering into what is truly a collaborative production. With a friend as donor, you may feel that your child can inherit your ethnicity though gestation, your donor's through genetics, your husband's through genetics—and celebrate all three.

Character, personality and intelligence

As with intrafamily donation, you will have to feel good about your donor's character and personality. She will be in your life and your child's life in some way, large or small, and you will want to like her very much. You'll want her to be someone you fully trust, admire and respect, and, with a friend, you have the advantage of a broad perspective when it comes to her intelligence. You've seen her in action and you know if she has common sense as opposed to "book smarts," emotional intelligence as opposed to high SAT scores. Knowing her, you feel capable of confirming that she is a capable person.

Cost

As with intrafamily donors, you save agency costs but incur all other costs. You won't be paying your friend a fee but you are likely to choose to give her a gift that is the equivalent in dollar terms of a donor fee. At the time of writing, payment of about $5000 in the US would seem appropriate.

Ethical considerations

In many ways, friend-to-friend donation reduces most ethical considerations in egg donation. Your donor is neither enticed by money nor obligated by family bonds. Most likely, she is making this donation free and clear of any form of coercion. You will want to do your best to make sure, however, that she fully understands all that is involved and that she still wants to donate after learning about the medical procedures, the child's possible future questions and so on.

Our family

As with any other donor, the composition of your existing family—nuclear and extended—will inform your thinking. If your husband has children and you do not, you may feel that having a friend as donor diminishes your role—"She's too visible, she's too present"—or you may feel it further authenticates you. You may feel more comfortable choosing a donor who no one knows, who you feel offers you some privacy and clearer family boundaries.

Special considerations

Here are some special considerations unique to friend and acquaintance donation.

FINDING YOUR DONOR

There are instances in which friends or acquaintances, aware of your infertility struggles, offer to donate their eggs. These lovely—and often unexpected offers—are unusual. Most often, someone hoping for a friend-to-friend donation must identify and seek their donor. How do you figure out who, among your many friends and acquaintances, might be a donor?

Once again, we turn to the idea of a letter. You might think of a few people you know who fit the bill and target them in a general letter that seems to be going to many people. You can write it in a broad-brushed way that doesn't put the person on the spot in any way. You might simply write:

> As you know, we have been struggling to have a baby. We've decided that our next step is egg donation and we are currently looking for someone who might be willing to donate eggs to us. We are looking for someone between ages __ and __ (you determine), who is in good physical and mental health, likes the idea of helping us

build our family and is willing and available to go through a time-consuming and sometimes uncomfortable medical process. If you have any friends who might consider this or if you might be willing to talk with us about donating, please let us know…

PRIVACY AND SECRECY

Most parents through egg donation believe in being open about the fact that they used donated eggs but want to maintain privacy about the donor's identity because they see it as their child's private information. How does one manage these privacy concerns when the donor is a friend? We know a happy mom through egg donation who is grateful to a co-worker for donating. Her family and friends all know she had a donor, but few know the identity of the donor. Both the recipient and the donor feel this is private and between them, but they are also aware that, in their efforts to maintain privacy, they have generated some sense of mystery around the donation. This is but one example of how issues of privacy and secrecy can arise in friend-to-friend donation.

IS THE OFFER SINCERE?

"I could do that. I'm happy to do that. You can have my eggs." The words are spoken. They come quickly and spontaneously, but are they real? Does the person who offered fully grasp what she has just said or will she want to rescind her offer?

Sometimes someone knows that a friend or acquaintance is looking for a donor and decides she wants to make an offer. She may do some research on egg donation and talk with people close to her about whether this is a good idea. Her offer is most likely sincere and made in an informed way. She might still change her mind when she goes to the medical program, but this is less likely to happen than when someone offers spontaneously, upon hearing of your struggles.

Program-recruited donors

Embarking on a search for a program-recruited donor is a strange and unfamiliar experience. Although some of you may locate your program donor in other ways, most of you will begin by looking at profiles online. How strange is that? Very strange, although less so for those of you who met your husbands or wives online. Whether it be Match.com or an egg donor agency website, online photos and profiles should serve as just the beginning of getting to know someone. Think of it as the first introduction, but know that more information can and should follow.

Which brings us to the question of how well you will come to know a donor you find through an agency or, perhaps, medical program. In some instances, very little. Programs in the Czech Republic, for example, insist on anonymity. You receive some information about your donor but no option of contact by email, phone, letter or in person. By contrast, programs in the US are increasingly aware of the many reasons why someone would want to meet their donor. As noted psychologist Elaine Gordon states:

> How can you "know" a donor or have gut sense of that individual if you have not actually met that person? To take it a bit further, who is the best person to select one's donor? It is the recipient. To choose a donor based on a few pictures and a profile is selling intended parents short. (Gordon 2011)

We would add to Dr. Gordon's caution by saying we feel it also sells the future child short. How strange would it be for a child, naturally curious, to ask questions to his parents about the donor and to hear, "We didn't meet her" or, worse still, "We don't know her name." Later in this section, we will address the question of when and how to meet your donor, but, first, to the task at hand: finding someone online.

So how do you begin to look at donors online? We suggest that you begin by limiting your search to perhaps four programs. A good donor can land anywhere, but you will drive yourself crazy if you hop from one site to the other and another. Instead, pick a few, based on ones your doctor feels comfortable working with, and begin your search. We expect that the first few times you go online you will feel bewildered.

We use the term *program-recruited donors* rather than anonymous donors because we don't feel that egg donors should remain anonymous. If you go to an agency, your donor will begin as a stranger, but, for a variety of reasons, we encourage you to bring her out of the shadows and into the daylight. Reasons for this include your comfort with who she is and why she is donating, building a story that will make sense for your child and ensuring you have some means of contact in the future.

Fertility

When people go to an agency seeking a donor, most assume she will be fertile. After all, she is being presented as a donor: why wouldn't she be fertile?

As we all know, pregnancy is the only guarantee of fertility: all else is a guess or a prediction. That said, one of the reasons people go to agencies to find donors is because many are proven donors, meaning they have donated before. If you select someone who has donated previously, you know that she took her medications correctly, responded well and, in most instances, you will receive non-identifying information about the number of embryos and whether a pregnancy occurred. If your donor has donated in your physician's practice, you have the added benefit of knowing that your practice knows what protocol works well with her.

Some women have donated several times. We will question this later from an ethical perspective, but, from the standpoint of fertility, this may not be a good thing. There are anecdotal reports of fertility/egg quality decreasing after several stimulated cycles.

The child's story

As with all donors, you will want to offer your child a story that he can understand, make sense of and feel good about. Surely your child will ask about this special woman who gave him life and you will want to be able to identify her by name, rather than a number, and, if possible, be able to describe her. If your donor is unwilling to meet you or if you are unable to meet her because of government or other regulations, be sure to gather as much information as you can about her. Remember, you are the first authors of your child's story and you want to write a story that will offer your child a strong, secure foundation to understanding how he came to be.

Appearance

If you are looking for a donor online, her appearance is likely the first thing that will prompt you to notice her. The photos she provides not only give you some sense of whether she resembles you physically, but they also provide some introduction to who she is as a person. What she is wearing, how she poses, the expression on her face, her smile, the look in her eyes will all influence your decision making. If you like what you see of her in the photos, you are likely to want to know more. Conversely, there may be a donor who looks quite a bit like you but you find yourself immediately turned off by a provocative pose, a foolish outfit or something else you see in a photo. After all, these are the photos she has *chosen* as her way of introducing herself to you.

Health

As we've said, everyone has some health issues in their family and almost no one takes a health history with everyone they date. We find ourselves suspicious of donor profiles with health histories that look "too good" and feel reassured that someone is telling the truth when she includes her mom's breast cancer or her grandfather's type 1 diabetes. As you review medical histories, we encourage you to be both true to yourself and open-minded. For example, I (Ellen) interviewed one couple in which the man had psoriasis that had plagued him all his life, and he and his wife felt very strongly about avoiding this condition in their donor. At the same time, however, they would accept a donor with other seemingly more serious conditions in her family because "these things happen."

In their 2009 study of 287 egg donors, Kramer, Schneider and Schultz report that 97.4 percent say they were never contacted by their donor agencies or medical programs for health updates, and 31 percent of the donors surveyed said that either they or close family members did indeed have medical issues arise that were important for families to know about. This study reminds us that a health intake form at the time of donation is but a snapshot in time of the donor's health. It is important to know what happens after that date.

Ethnicity

For some of you, finding a donor who shares your ethnic background is essential, especially if your donor begins as a stranger. You may be someone who would have been okay having a close friend donate even if she was of a different ethnic group. However, with program-recruited donors, the fact that a woman shares your ethnicity can make her seem more familiar, can help take the process away from the sci-fi realm and into real life. You don't know her, but she's Italian and you are Italian and so you feel a connection.

In looking at countless profiles online, we have seen that the vast majority of donors are of mixed ethnicity. You may be full Irish or full Italian or Greek and discover that it is hard to find your ethnic match online. Perhaps this has to do with geography: some areas have a higher representation of one ethnic group over another. In addition, as the rate of intermarriage—of all sorts—increases, there are more and more younger people of mixed ethnicity. The donors you are considering may be ten or more years younger than you and hence more likely to have parents from different ethnic or racial groups. We have found that many recipients who embark upon their donor search hoping for a full ethnic match content themselves, along the way, with someone who shares some portion of their ethnicity.

Character, personality and intelligence

Just as photos tell you a lot about the donors you "meet" online, so also does the profile. Her responses to questions ranging from "Who is the person you most admire?" to "What is your favorite childhood memory?" give you some sense of who she is as a person, how she sees herself, what her values are and how she reacts to the world around her. We all know that someone can write what they think you want to read and sometimes these canned replies are easy to identify. At the same time as there are some predictable responses, there are many donors who write beautiful, poignant paragraphs about their families, their friends, their formative life experiences. It is common for recipients to feel that they "know" someone after reading her profile. It is also common to be particularly moved by one comment or observation the donor writes.

Unfortunately, donor agencies have no standardized questionnaire. Each has its own form and format, and some, we find, are much easier to read than others. Although there are some questions that tend to be on all questionnaires—such as "Why do you want to donate?"—other questions vary from one form to another. We have been struck by how little the questionnaires ask donors about their feelings about donating, about the family they hope to help and about the child they hope to help bring into the world. Odd, it seems, that questions such as "Do you believe in miracles?" and "What is your favorite color?" are more prevalent.

As we said earlier, we see the online questionnaires as a beginning introduction and agree with Dr. Elaine Gordon when she stresses the importance of meeting the donor. At the same time, however, we know that many of you *will* be basing your decision on what you read online. We encourage you to feel that you can ask the donor agency for the answers to further questions you may pose or request additional photos. You need, however it happens, to feel very good about your donor, especially with regard to her character and personality.

Intelligence, as we noted in earlier sections, can take many forms. If you know your donor, you can make your own assessment about her intelligence. When you are relying on online profiles, you will be more likely to look for what seems to be objective evidence of her intelligence: what college did she attend, what was her grade point average, her standardized test scores? We encourage you to look beyond these bits of information, as best you can, and at the full picture, as people's life circumstances will so often influence where they attend college or how high their grades are. Instead, you might want to make decisions based on what she is doing with her life, what goals she is setting for herself, how realistic these goals seem to be and how is she going about trying to achieve them.

Cost

As you look at donor agencies and profiles, you will see that the costs vary from one agency to another and that donor fees sometimes vary from donor to donor. When you consider agency fees, look carefully so that you know you are comparing apples with apples. Fees may be broken down in various ways, but what matters is the bottom line: what will it cost you to work with this agency? The other thing you will surely want to know is what fees might you incur if your donor falls through and you want to choose a donor from another agency. Will the money you have paid this agency be reimbursed in full or in part?

The other cost to consider is your donor's fee. This ties in to our next topic of ethical considerations. If we assume that you prefer to choose a donor who is not motivated primarily by payment, then the fee she is requesting is significant. Some programs have one fee for all donors, something we strongly prefer, but many programs allow/encourage donors to raise their fees when they are proven donors. We don't exactly get this reasoning since, according to the American Society for Reproductive Medicine, fees to donors are for time and effort and not payment for eggs. If this is the case, why would someone's time and effort increase in a second donation? There may be unusual circumstances, such as a second donation requiring more travel, but, in most instances, someone spends less time focused on an egg donor cycle, rather than more, when they have donated before.

Ethical considerations

If we assume that you want to choose a donor who is making a decision that is right for her, as well as right for you and your hoped-for child, then you will want someone who you feel has truly achieved informed consent. Some might argue that no young woman can really know how she will feel in the future when she looks back on her decision to donate, but there are certain features of her current circumstances that suggest someone being better able—or less able—to have informed consent. These include:

1. Does she have children? Although many program-recruited donors do not have children, some do. A woman who is already a mom knows what kinship means to her and seems to be in a better position to know what she is giving up when she donates eggs.

2. How did she become involved in egg donation? You may not learn what prompted her to donate from the questionnaire, but some donors will volunteer this information. I (Ellen) had one client who chose a donor who is a nurse in an infertility clinic and wrote that she decided to donate when she came to see the pain of infertility. Another donor's mother had twins through egg donation and the donor, their older half-sister, wanted to give back. Another donor is a single mother through sperm donation who also wanted to give back.

3. Although some young women are wise and experienced beyond their years, chronological age counts. We wonder if a young woman under the age of 23 or 24 can anticipate how she will feel years hence knowing a part of her is "out in the world."

4. If we assume that your hoped-for child will be curious about the donor, her children, her future children and her nieces and nephews, is she someone who will agree to be available to you and your family, if not through direct contact then through the Donor Sibling Registry?

Another ethical consideration involves donor anonymity. Even if you agree with us that it is problematic to have a donor who is and will remain anonymous, the reality is that many program-recruited donors are still anonymous. What do you do if the donor you want—because she looks like you and seems to be a really good person and shares your ethnic heritage—is someone who wants to remain anonymous? You can ask your agency to talk with her and try to determine if this preference is written in stone or if she feels she can be flexible. We have found that it is not uncommon for the donor to respond that she is willing to be available to the child in the future but does not want to meet you now. If this is her response, you might conclude that it is good enough, in that you have successfully addressed your primary ethical concern: that your child not be cut off from his genetic heritage.

Donors and recipients who recognize the benefits of contact but want to maintain anonymity are turning to the Donor Sibling Registry (DSR) in increasing numbers. At the time of writing, Wendy Kramer, DSR director, reports that increasing numbers of donor agencies and medical programs are assisting clients by including the DSR in their donor–recipient legal agreements. When a baby is born, he is registered on the DSR so that the donor and recipient have a means in place to communicate with each other. Kramer observes people using the DSR to send medical updates, social updates and photos.

Although she is pleased that donors and recipients who choose anonymity can use the DSR to be in contact, Kramer believes that it would be better for all involved to have direct contact. She notes that 77 percent of the 751 donor offspring that she surveyed recommend that their parents use non-anonymous donors. When she surveyed 108 egg donor parents and asked them if they wished they had an open/identity or known donor, 49.3 percent said yes. When asked why they did not originally choose open donors, nearly 70 percent said their clinics did not make open/identity donors available and over 10 percent said they didn't even know open donors existed.

Our family

Your family members—older children, your parents, siblings—will surely be curious about the "stranger" you find to be your donor. How much or how little do you share about her? On the one hand, we have known recipients who felt strongly about having close family members share in their process of donor selection: it felt comforting to have their mother or sister review profiles with them. Others treat the donor's identity as the child's private information and conclude that family members should know only that you found a donor, you feel really good about her and you feel great about your decision to take this path.

Because egg donation is becoming increasingly common, it is no longer unusual for a recipient to have a family member who has also become a parent through egg donation. While this can be nice for the children and something special for the sisters to share, it can also be problematic. I (Ellen) have a client going through egg donation whose sister recently had a baby through anonymous donation. She plans to tell very few people how her child came to be. My client plans to meet her donor and be open with her child about the donor's identity and quite open with others about egg donation in general. The two sisters' different approaches to parenthood through egg donation are prompting some conflict between them.

Special considerations

If you are thinking of program-recruited donation, here are some special considerations unique to program-recruited donation.

MEETING YOUR DONOR

Although we encourage you to meet your donor at some point, assuming that you live in a country and are working with a program that allows this, we're aware that, for many recipients, it is difficult to meet prior to pregnancy. For some, this may be a matter of logistics and geography, but, for many others, you simply feel too vulnerable. Too much has gone wrong for you to feel that you can risk meeting someone, liking her a lot and then facing more disappointment if she does not produce eggs, if fertilization is poor or if you don't become pregnant or you miscarry. For all of these reasons, many recipients feel more comfortable postponing a meeting until a pregnancy is well established or, even safer still, until a child has been born. In addition, some donors also prefer to meet after the fact as a later meeting spares them any sense that they are being evaluated or judged.

As we see it, the important decision is *to meet* your donor; *when* this happens is of less consequence. Meeting in advance offers the comfort of a truly collaborative effort and promotes a sense that your donor is your partner in this intimate endeavor, not some distant shadowy figure. Some recipients have said that they felt more confident that it would work once they met their donor. But, as we acknowledged earlier, you may feel too vulnerable, after all you have been through, to meet her in advance.

So where should the meeting occur, whether it be before or after a cycle? I (Ellen) have known donors and recipients who exchanged emails and phone numbers and agreed to meet in a Starbucks or a deli. One woman arrived at the deli early, gave the server a large advanced tip and asked that she take a photo of her and the woman she would be with.

Many recipients and donors feel more comfortable meeting with a counselor or some other facilitator. I (Ellen) have facilitated a number of these meetings and have found them to be remarkably similar. For one thing, intended/expectant/new moms often prefer to meet their donor on their own, without their husband or partner. They explain this feeling by saying, "It's between two women." Regardless of who attends, I've found that participants are usually anxious at first, but their anxiety melts away within moments of meeting each other. The meetings, which have usually lasted about 45 minutes, have been filled with a lively, warm conversation about their lives. I always tell participants to feel free to ask each other anything, but that each should feel equally free to say that something feels too private or that they'd prefer not to talk about it.

Donor siblings and cousins

All these are reasons for you and your donor to participate in the Donor Sibling Registry but if she is unwilling or unable to do so for any reason, there are some things you can do in beginning the process that might prove helpful down the line. If your donor is someone who has donated before or will donate in the future, has children of her own or will have them in the future, you are likely to have thoughts and feelings about who else your child could be related to. In addition, if the donor has siblings and they, at any point, have children, these children will be genetic first cousins.

1. Find out how many siblings she has and if they already have children. Some of this will be on your donor's profile.

2. Pay attention to the age and gender of any children your donor has.

3. Learn about any other donor cycles she might have had. Where did she donate? Did a singleton or twin pregnancy occur? Ask if your donor or agency will notify you of future cycles. We realize that this may sound bold and that your agency or physician may well tell you this information is not your concern, but ask a donor-conceived adult if these questions matter and they will most likely confirm the importance of knowing all they can about donor "siblings" and "cousins." It is there as a resource for your child, but we believe your child will appreciate knowing that you anticipated questions he might have and did your best at the start to find answers.

Donor banks

Women seeking egg donation can now access donors through egg banks. This route is sometimes attractive to recipients who have had donors fall through or who cannot afford the often higher costs of other forms of egg donation. Some weary travelers like the fact that, with an egg bank, the donor has already followed through with her donation and the eggs are there. Egg banks also generally offer some guarantee of the number of eggs recipients will receive.

Because we approach egg donation from the perspectives of acting in the best interest of children and building family stories that all members feel comfortable with, we have major concerns about egg banks. For one thing, they promote anonymity. The website of My Egg Bank North America, a prominent egg bank located in Atlanta, Georgia, says that all donors are anonymous and notes that they will not even share adult photos with recipients. Having heard from sperm-donor offspring of the consequences of anonymity, we worry how donor-bank offspring will feel about their origins. In addition, we wonder how loving parents will share this story. It is one thing to tell a child that a sister or close friend donated or that you found a very special woman whom you came to know and trust to help you have a baby. That seems different from saying that you went to a bank where women deposit eggs for others to use in the future. In other words, the bank seems to remove the human connection between two women. Social worker, Susan Levin, has interviewed several women donating to egg banks as well as couples seeking their donors through banks. She notes that the donors do have feelings about the families they are helping to build and that the intended parents are finding ways to build a family story that they feel good about. Levin encourages them to focus the story on how they came together as a family rather than on the specifics of the donor, noting, "It's not just about the information—it's about how you tell it and most important, that you feel it was a good decision for you."

If you are making decisions about how and where you will find your donor, if you are making decisions about how and where you will find your donor, turning to an egg bank may prove to be the right option for you. If it is, there may be information you can secure from the egg bank that will enable your child to work with the Donor Sibling Registry or find some other means of accessing his donor (and donor siblings) in the future.

Shelley, Allison, Jenna and Grace, mothers all

We have talked about the various kinds of donors and the advantages and disadvantages you might encounter with each. What we want to leave you with is the *good* news: people *do* find donors that are *right* for them and egg donation often works. We'd like to take a moment to introduce you to Shelley, Allison, Jenna and Grace. Four different women. Four different donors. Four happy mothers.

Shelley was born in the former Soviet Union. She and her family came to the US when she was 13, right around the time that she learned that she had no ovarian function. The doctors speculated that she might have been a victim of fallout from Chernobyl. In any event, Shelley spent many years believing that she would never have a baby. When she was in her late 20s, her younger sister, Natalie, read an article on egg donation and came to her, offering to help. Shelley was stunned by her offer. An educated woman, she had purposefully avoided reading anything about assisted reproduction because it was simply too painful. She had managed, somehow, to miss that egg donation was an option for her and she certainly had no idea that her sister, a few years younger than her, would be willing and able to donate. Shelley has a three-year-old daughter, Missy, and plans to undergo an embryo transfer, from the cycle that brought her Missy, in coming months.

Allison really didn't like the idea of egg donation. She had siblings who were adopted, and when she and her husband encountered infertility, Allison felt certain they would adopt. Then along came Megan, a colleague at work with the words, "I'll donate." Allison did not take this offer seriously at first, but Megan brought it up again. And again. Over time it became clear that Megan was truly committed to donating to Allison. Although reluctant and not at all sure egg donation was right for them, Allison proceeded. To her surprise, after years in which every pregnancy effort resulted in disappointment, all went well. Megan produced several eggs, fertilization was good and, to Allison's shock and disbelief, she became pregnant. Initially, Allison was not overjoyed at being pregnant—she felt sad and angry that Megan's eggs had worked and hers had not. However, this changed over time, and as her unborn child grew inside her, Allison's joy trumped her feelings of loss. Holding her baby for the first time, Allison, who endured a three-day labor that ended in a C-section, was all smiles—and tears. "I can't begin to say thank you to Megan. She changed my life and that of my family forever." Then she added, "If I ever have another child, I want to do it the very same way."

Jenna became pregnant when she was 40 and for the first few weeks all seemed to be going so well. Jenna felt that her luck had changed and that, after several years, she and Brad would finally have a baby. Then came the amnio and the news that the fetus she was carrying had Down syndrome. Jenna and Brad made the decision to terminate the pregnancy, an experience that was devastating to them in so many ways. In the weeks that followed the procedure, Jenna often felt that she would never smile again. Then a close friend had a baby through egg donation and coaxed Jenna to think about this option. Reluctantly, Jenna went online and began slowly looking at donors. From the sea of online faces emerged Sonia, a 27-year-old mother of two young children who had donated to a close friend, felt good about the experience and now wanted to help a childless couple. Although she had hoped for a local donor and Sonia lived across the country, Jenna was certain she had found her donor. She made arrangements through the donor agency and her medical program to bring Sonia to Providence, Rhode Island, where Jenna lives. Sonia came graciously. The two women met while Sonia was approaching retrieval. A little more than two weeks later, Jenna received a positive pregnancy test and soon discovered that she was having twins.

Like many women, Grace came reluctantly to egg donation. There were many things she didn't like about it and one was the anonymity of many donors. Grace spoke to her sister about this and her sister, a nurse, told her that one of her colleagues, a lovely young woman, had been thinking about donating eggs. "Maybe she will donate to you. You could get to know her and that might go a long way towards making you feel more comfortable with egg donation." Indeed it did. Susanna, the donor, traveled to Massachusetts to meet Grace and the two women hit it off. They agreed to proceed with a donor cycle and, a few months later, Susanna returned for the donation. The cycle went well and yielded many eggs, most of which fertilized. Grace had one transferred and learned two weeks later that she was pregnant. To everyone's surprise, she was carrying twins. The embryo had split and Grace was pregnant with monozygotic twins. Sadly, she lost the twins at eight weeks, a loss that was devastating but not wholly unexpected as this form of identical twins is difficult to carry. Grace returned for three frozen embryo transfer cycles, none of which resulted in pregnancy. Depleted of energy and money, Grace and her husband, Jack, decided it was time to give up—to accept that they would not have children. Then Grace learned that egg banks were now an option. "I need to give it this one last try," she declared. "I'm going to Atlanta." Nine months later, Grace delivered baby Noah.

Four different women. Mothers all.

– 5 –

Mental Health Counseling and Legal Issues

"The people you meet along the way shape your journey." This is one of the central themes of this book, and it is especially relevant to this chapter. Whether you use a relative or acquaintance as your donor or use a program-recruited donor found through a medical clinic or commercial program, you will surely meet and use mental health counselors and lawyers as you make plans to attempt pregnancy through egg donation. Their roles are distinct and very different, but individuals in each category of "helping people" play significant roles in an egg donation journey.

Egg donation and mental health counselors

First, a word about titles. We are identifying those who can counsel you about the emotional aspects of egg donation with the umbrella label of "mental health counselor." The reason for this is that mental health professionals working in the field of infertility come from a range of backgrounds. They may be psychiatrists, psychologists, social workers or psychiatric nurses. In certain instances, it may be helpful for that person to be a psychiatrist or a psychiatric nurse practitioner, since they can help you make any decisions about psychiatric medications. Similarly, there are instances in which the skills of a psychologist—someone skilled in psychological testing—are called for. However, what matters for most people considering egg donation is that the mental health counselor(s) they speak with be well versed in the medical and psychological experience of infertility.

Women and men considering egg donation meet with mental health counselors for one of two reasons: the individual or couple proactively seeks counseling or the individual or couple is instructed to see a counselor by their egg donor program. Either way, you should identify someone who is knowledgeable about egg donation. Counselors specializing in this area can be located through national or regional fertility organizations, through your medical program and, often most helpful, by referral from another infertility patient.

We are using the word "counseling" and not "psychotherapy" intentionally. In most instances, what you will be doing with a counselor will have very little to do with the distant past. Surely there are instances in which infertility resonates with someone's early life experiences and there may be a benefit in psychotherapy, but, for the most part, we are suggesting a present- and future-oriented counseling that, in many ways, resembles coaching. In fact, I (Ellen) often identify myself as a fertility coach, as do some of my colleagues.

When counseling is required

Although many people seek help from a counselor while they are in the throes of infertility treatment or perhaps following a miscarriage, there are some who do not. If you are someone who feels "I can handle things on my own," or who is otherwise disinclined to use counseling or psychotherapy, you may be surprised when your medical program instructs you to see someone. You may even be a bit put off or offended, wondering if your physician or nurse is somehow questioning your stability.

So why does a medical program require someone to see a counselor? Most professionals working with egg donation are aware that any type of collaborative reproduction involves complex ethical issues for both donor and recipient. Sometimes a patient lets the medical staff know that they are having a hard time. Perhaps you are calling the nurses frequently and expressing a great deal of anxiety. Possibly, you are telling them of stress in your marriage or with your family or your job. Contacts like these may prompt staff to suggest to you that you talk with a counselor. Occasionally, a patient's upset or anxiety is so pronounced that counseling is required before moving forward with treatment.

In most instances, a recommendation of counseling is not a commentary on your stability. Many programs require everyone going through assisted reproduction to have at least one meeting with a counselor. Counseling is most often mandated because you are undergoing a particular form of assisted reproductive technology. Many centers require one counseling session for third-party reproduction. In instances of known donation—a family member or friend—there will probably be a series of required visits.

We know that most people don't like to be told what to do and that being instructed to see a counselor can feel paternalistic or judgmental. I (Ellen) can only say that there have been countless times when people sent to me have ended the session by saying, "I'm so glad we were required to do this—it was so helpful" or "I wish I had spoken with you earlier in this process." My sense is that many people are relieved to talk with someone who is very familiar with what they are going through, has information to provide and understands things from an emotional perspective. It can also be reassuring to have someone you can call in the future, should you have questions or concerns that could be addressed in counseling.

The sequence and format of this counseling will vary, but the following are issues that should be addressed in counseling before you enter an egg donation cycle.

Volunteer known donor

If you are working with a family member or friend, you will probably be asked to participate in a series of meetings. The first meeting may be with the donor alone, it may be with you (and your partner) or it may include both donor and recipients. Some counselors prefer to meet with the prospective donor first so they can help her make the best decision for herself. This may include helping give her an "out" if donation is not right for her at this time. Counselors who see the donor first feel this helps them as counselors to avoid feeling any obligation to the recipients. Other counselors prefer to meet with the recipients first in order to have some sense of history and a perspective on how this came about. These counselors feel they can remain open to helping a donor say no, if she feels she wants or needs to do so.

Regardless of who is seen first, the role of the counselor in meeting with recipients and with their volunteer donors is to try to confirm that everyone is entering into this with comfort and shared expectations. If the counselor senses that any participant (and this could be the donor's husband/partner) is uncomfortable with the endeavor, it is the counselor's responsibility to help the uneasy participant out of their dilemma. This assistance may take the form of additional counseling—to help participants either feel more comfortable with their decision or to make an alternative plan.

Whether you are going forward with your volunteer donor or moving on to some other option, there should be at least one visit that includes both couples (assuming the donor has a partner). This visit could address potential reasons not to move forward, or, more likely, it will be an opportunity to solidify your plans together. Assuming the latter, the visit will be a time during which all participants can discuss their expectations for their relationships in the future and, specifically, their relationships with regard to the child or children that may result from the donation. It will also be important to talk about the possibility of disappointment—donors and recipients may do their best and still not achieve a successful pregnancy.

A conjoint meeting with a counselor will also provide everyone with a foundation for counseling in the future, should any or all of you need to talk again. Something could come up either during a cycle, during a pregnancy or after the birth of a child that you will want to discuss with someone who knows the history of the donation.

PROGRAM-RECRUITED DONOR

If you are working with a program-recruited donor and have no plans to meet her, you may be asked to have only one session with a counselor. This session can assist you in donor selection, if that is something you have not already done on your own, or it can focus on your feelings about the donor you have chosen. The session can address any issues a couple may have that might get in the way during a cycle, during pregnancy or later.

If you plan to meet your donor, the counseling session can help you plan for and anticipate this meeting. The counselor can assist you in deciding whether you want to meet your donor prior to a cycle or some time later. She can serve as a sounding board if you are still struggling with uncertainty about which donor to pick and can help you as you grapple with the reality that there is no absolute "right" or "wrong" donor. You will be drawn to one woman for a particular reason and to another for a different reason. What matters is that you settle on a donor, feel good about your decision and feel optimistic as you move forward.

If you are meeting your donor, you may want to have a counselor participate in the meeting. Although many people describe wonderful meetings that occur with their donors at Starbucks or a local diner or deli, there are some advantages to having a counselor at your meeting. In addition to being there to make introductions and to smooth over any awkward silences, she can play an important role in helping you and your donor feel comfortable raising questions. I (Ellen) always begin donor-recipient meetings by encouraging each participant to feel free to ask questions but to know that the other participant(s) may not want to respond. I encourage people to feel that privacy is respected but urge them not to censor themselves unnecessarily. A practical reason for having a counselor be part of the meeting is that she can help you figure out when to end it and, if you want, take a photo of the two/three of you together.

Seeking help proactively

People considering or participating in egg donation seek help from a counselor for a variety of reasons. The following are among the most common issues experienced by egg donor couples.

LOSS AND GRIEF

No one gets to advanced infertility treatment without experiencing loss. Your losses may have occurred years ago, perhaps when you were a young adult facing cancer treatment or recovering from emergency surgery that removed your ovaries. Or your losses were more recent—you tried to conceive, never anticipating a problem, and learned that you had premature ovarian failure. Possibly, you are one of the many people who always wanted to have a baby but didn't find a partner until your eggs were "too old." Or you may have experienced pregnancy loss, maybe even the devastation of a late loss or a loss of twins or triplets. Whatever the nature of your loss, it has to be there as part of what you carry with you as you move forward.

A mental health counselor can assist you with your feelings of loss and grief, and prevent them from interfering with the joy of parenthood through egg donation. Counseling can offer you the opportunity to talk about what you have been through, what it meant to you to have your own biological child and what it means to move forward with egg donation, knowing that a part of you will always ache.

Issues of loss and grief will differ depending upon whether you have had a biological child, whether you always knew you couldn't reproduce, whether you are filled with regret (e.g. for delaying parenthood) or with gratitude that this option exists. The loss of a child that existed only in your hopes and dreams is a form of disenfranchised loss—one for which there are no rituals of mourning. A counselor can assist you in creating your own rituals. For example, you may choose to write a letter to the child you never had or plant a tree.

A counselor can help you find a way to accept that your sorrow and your joy can sit side by side. If you conceive through the help of an egg donor, you will most likely be thrilled, but you may also feel some sadness about what is not to be. Mental health counselors have found that those couples who most fully acknowledge their loss and grief over not having a full biological child (or a second) are often more prepared to enjoy and embrace egg donation fully. One couple who turned to egg donation after years of infertility and was now expecting their first baby captured the combination of emotions when they said, "We're 'over the top happy' and yet it is still very sad. We feel there has been a death in the family, but we are moving on with such joy and so much hope."

DECISION MAKING

Your journey to parenthood has been a complicated one and it is not over yet. As you consider egg donation, there are decisions to be made. Is this the right option for you? If so, what type of donor do you prefer—family, friend, anonymous? How can you ask someone to donate? How do you select a program-recruited donor? Will you meet her? If so, should you wait until you are pregnant or meet her in advance? Would you prefer to talk with her by phone rather than meet face to face? If egg donation does not work, will you turn to adoption or, possibly, to combining egg donation with a gestational carrier? Or will you choose not to have children, or, in instances of secondary infertility, not to expand your family? A counselor knowledgeable about various paths to parenthood and the psychological processes involved in pursuing them can help you sort through these decisions and others that may arise.

RELATIONSHIP ISSUES

Many people considering egg donation are part of a couple, either heterosexual or same-sex. All couples face incredible challenges figuring out how to keep their relationship strong while undergoing procedures that are stressful, intrusive, sometimes physically painful and of uncertain outcome. Couples rarely move at the same pace through infertility treatment and egg donation, and they don't always agree about second-choice paths to parenthood. Even those who do agree on what to do and when to do it may face differences about where to seek treatment, how long to try a particular approach and, in the case of egg donation, which program to use and which donor. Additional areas of potential conflict include differences about who to talk with about egg donation, what to say and when to say it.

Couples work hard to share egg donation, but some still feel that they have unequal roles. Women who feel that genetic ties are more important than gestational bonds may enter into the process still feeling envy of their husbands and, perhaps, a sense of unfairness. You may feel that you were beyond this and were ready to fully embrace motherhood through egg donation, but now you are tired, nauseous and feeling that your body is being taken over. It may all feel very unfair. Your husband or partner gets to have his biological child and you get to do all the work. Counselors serve as objective intermediaries in helping couples work through such differences.

Couples undergoing infertility and those pursuing egg donation or other options often find it helpful to have a counselor who can accompany them on their journey. Couples counseling for infertility, like individual counseling in this area, need not be weekly or even every second week. Rather, it can be helpful to know someone over time—to have her or him there and available as a resource. This counselor can help you listen more clearly to each other, avoiding such common Achilles' heels of infertile couples as hearing "not yet" as "never," believing there is no potential for compromise and feeling that one's partner either wants to talk about infertility all the time or never at all.

Relationships with family, friends and helping professionals

Pursuing egg donation usually involves juggling a variety of relationships. You will be making decisions about what you say to family members and friends—whether you tell them you are choosing egg donation, whether you share information about the donor, whether you decide to wait until after you are pregnant or after you have your baby or later. You will also be navigating relationships with caregivers, some of whom may be responsive and sensitive to your feelings and others who may seem always to miss the boat.

A mental health counselor can help you sort through your reactions to and interactions with the cast of characters in your life. Someone who has talked with countless others facing similar struggles will understand what you go through when you learn your little sister is pregnant, when you are invited to yet another baby shower, when your cousin says something disparaging about egg donation, or when your mother tells you to "just adopt." The counselor can assist you in preparing for your conversations with people at work, with your physicians and with prospective egg donors, whether they are family members, friends or strangers.

Preparing for egg donation

Many of you have been through IVF or some other high-tech intervention before arriving at egg donation. Chances are that you also feel experienced with the procedures and therefore prepared for a donor egg cycle. What you may not have anticipated are the ways that this process can feel different from earlier treatment regimens. A counselor can help you prepare for any and all of the following.

DONOR SELECTION

Selecting a donor can feel like an enormous responsibility. If you are deciding whether to work with a family member or friend, you will probably be grappling with questions about what it will mean to your relationship with that individual as well as with other family members or friends. You will also be wondering if your volunteer donor really wants to do this or whether she feels pressured or coerced. A counselor can help you explore your feelings about having someone close to you donate and she can be available to meet with your donor to help confirm that the decision is right for all participants.

If you seek a program-recruited donor, you will most likely feel a great responsibility to "get it right." People play out this feeling in a variety of ways. Some conclude that they've got it right because they feel a powerful chemistry with the donor. Others attempt to get it right by carefully scrutinizing the donor's photos, SAT scores and interests in an effort to select the best genes.

> Mary, 35 and deciding between her sister and a contractual donor, put it this way: "If my sister donates, we get what we get. I know who she is and I'm going into this assuming the child will inherit some of her characteristics. But if we go with someone we find on a list of donors, it will be my responsibility to pick wisely. It feels like too much control. What if I make a mistake?"

A counselor can help you sort through your feelings about different donors and she can help you make your way through donor profiles. She can reflect your reactions back to you and help you gain confidence in your ability to make a good decision. She can also help you keep the burden of this decision in perspective, reminding you that no one really has control of who their child will be.

FEELINGS ABOUT WHAT THE DONOR—WHETHER KNOWN OR ANONYMOUS—IS GOING THROUGH

People whose sister or cousin or friend is donating are often worried about "what we are putting her through." However, you are not the only ones concerned about the well-being of your donor. Couples working with program-recruited donors also find themselves concerned about their donor, both during the time she is taking the medications and especially during egg retrieval. A counselor is available to meet with your known or unknown donor, help her resolve her own feelings and reassure you that her emotional needs are being met and that her feelings are normal and healthy.

AMBIVALENCE ABOUT THIS DECISION

Ambivalence will be your traveling companion throughout this journey and will, most likely, accompany you into parenthood. When you work so hard to make a decision and come to believe in the rightness of that decision, it can be terribly upsetting to encounter a resurgence of ambivalence. We hope you will feel comforted by a counselor who accepts your ambivalence and lets you know "it goes with the territory."

LOSS AND SELF-BLAME IF IT DOESN'T WORK

Couples work very hard to decide on egg donation, usually assuming that it will work. When a cycle fails or a miscarriage occurs, it is devastating. This devastation is often worse for a woman. You may feel it is the ultimate proof that your body does not work or, worse still, that you are "not meant to be a mother." You, who worked hard to move beyond the loss and self-blame that you felt prior to egg donation, may feel catapulted back to that painful state. A skilled counselor can be invaluable in helping you deal with this renewed grief.

ANXIETY AND DISBELIEF IF THE PREGNANCY TEST IS POSITIVE

It helps to be prepared for the strong possibility that you will be flooded with anxiety and disbelief if the pregnancy test is positive. The anxiety will be about loss and, perhaps, about fears that you've made a mistake or that there is something wrong with the baby. After all that you have been through to achieve an egg donation pregnancy, it is almost inevitable that you will have a complicated and, perhaps, inconsistent reaction to the news that you—or your wife/partner—are pregnant.

THE BLESSING AND CURSE OF THE MEANT TO BE

As we noted in our introduction, people experiencing infertility, pregnancy loss and third-party parenting often encounter the declaration "It was meant to be." While the words can be comforting when you have a wonderful baby through egg donation and cannot imagine loving any other child as much, they can sting when things do not go well. A pregnancy loss that was "not meant to be" can prompt you to feel that you forced nature. Although "it wasn't meant to be" can be a curse to anyone undergoing infertility, it carries with it special sting for those who turned reluctantly and with ethical, moral and religious questions to egg donation. Sensitive professional support can assist with this.

PREPARATION FOR TALKING WITH CHILDREN
Sadly, many parents through egg donation are afraid they won't be able to talk truthfully with their children. Specifically, they fear talking with their children about donor conception. An otherwise happy story—of a child wanted and planned for and loved—risks being transformed into a story of sadness and shame.

Your counselor can help you feel confident and prepared for future conversations. Before a cycle, it may be difficult to imagine you will ever become pregnant, let alone actually be a parent, so these practice conversations may seem remote. However, for many future parents, it is helpful to begin contemplating these conversations before pregnancy.

Group counseling
Groups can be especially helpful to people considering or pursuing egg donation and for those who are already parents through this process. Unlike adoptive parents, who may easily locate one another, either because they adopted transracially or because they met at an adoption agency or adoption organization, parents through egg donation have no easy ways of finding one another.

Joining a support group that introduces you to others who are parents through egg donation—or intended parents—will not only diminish your isolation; it will also provide you with valuable information as people will share their experiences with different medical and egg donation programs, as well as their experiences talking with others and with their children about egg donation.

Egg donation and the law

In egg donation, as in many areas of life involving legal relationships, lawyers have two types of roles: one is to try to prevent problems; the second is to step in when problems arise. We hope (and assume) your need for a lawyer familiar with egg donation will be limited to the first role, but we will provide you with information about the second as well.

Do I need an attorney?

Absolutely! To avoid legal conflicts related to egg donation, it is essential that all participants in the process seek their own legal counsel. By all participants, we mean not only the donors and recipients but also their medical and egg donation programs. Lawyers ensure that any agreements entered into are carefully drafted to comply with state and federal laws and avoid any confusion or misinterpretation regarding the rights, responsibilities or intent of all parties.

While an attorney is not always officially required by egg donor programs, egg donation is one of the most important undertakings a couple will ever consider. Due to its very nature, there are risks associated with egg donation, such as potential for disease, genetic disclosure, informed consent of medical risk and maternity determination, as well as ensuring that the egg donor is in no way exploited, just to name a few. In other words, while you do not legally need an attorney, it is wise for both donors and recipients to consult one.

What will a lawyer do?

In the US, there are only a few states that have statutes specifically dealing with egg donation. Lawyers advise that recipient couples and their donors—whether known or anonymous—enter into a legal agreement regarding all aspects of the donation. The intended parents should be represented by one lawyer and the donor by her own independent attorney. These contracts will address a range of matters including clearly defining the child's parentage, identifying the specific medical procedures to be undertaken, acknowledging the risks involved, making a genetic disclaimer and specifying plans for disposition of additional embryos. The contract should also detail when the eggs cease to belong to the donor and who controls the disposition of cryopreserved embryos now and in the future.

Another goal of the egg donation agreement is to establish the parties' intent that the resulting child or children will be the legal children of the biological father and the intended mother. Egg donor arrangements do not require either court involvement or a formal adoption, but the agreement will establish that the donor is relinquishing all parental rights for any child who is conceived through the donated eggs.

The written egg donation agreement should provide protection to all parties against claims brought by the other party for complications resulting from the egg donation procedure. Risks should be identified and allocated fairly. Ideally, insurance is available and purchased by the recipients for any medical complications. For example, the donor could claim damages for illness or injury during the donor cycle or even for emotional harm following donation. Similarly, without a written agreement concerning these issues, the intended parents could claim damages for complications during pregnancy or for genetic or congenital defects in the child.

In addition to providing certain safeguards, lawyers note that the process of negotiating a formal written agreement often serves to raise issues that the participants may not have fully considered. It is preferable for these issues to arise prior to the egg donation process rather than during a cycle or, worse still, during a pregnancy. If the participants cannot reach agreement on any sticking points, it usually makes sense for the intended parents to seek a new donor (or vice versa).

What should be included in a contract?

Because the laws regarding egg donation vary from one country to another and, in the US, from one state to another, it is difficult to provide a comprehensive summary of what should be included in an egg donation contract. The following are central issues usually covered in cotracts in the US.

- Identification of the parties involved. It is important to clearly identify each of the participants by role. For example, a contract may say, the "mother/recipient" and then explain she is "the woman who shall carry the child and ultimately be deemed its 'mother.'"

- Establishment of maternity and paternity. The contract should clearly establish who will be the parents of the child, spelling out that it is the mother/recipient and her husband (in the case of married, heterosexual couples) who will be the child's parents.

- Relinquishment of the donor's possible rights. Since in most instances it is the genetic mother and father of a child who have parental rights and this is not the case in egg donation, the contract should include a relinquishment of the donor's rights.

- Establishment of procedures to be undertaken. The contract should outline all of the medical screening, psychological screening, counseling and medical procedures that will be involved in egg donation, including ovulation induction, egg retrieval and embryo transfer.

- Risks. The contract should identify the short- and long-term medical and psychological risks associated with egg donation for all participants.

- Genetic disclaimer. The contract should indicate that certain diseases or conditions may be known to exist in the donor's family or may be found within certain populations or ethnic groupings. These conditions should be divulged and the risks assumed by the recipient couple. In order to assist the attending physicians of the child or children to be born, the medical and genetic history of the donor and donor's relatives should be provided by the egg donor.

- Embryo storage. The contract should specify whether embryos will be cryopreserved and, if so, where they will be stored, at what cost and to whom, and for what duration. It should also confirm that the cryopreserved embryos are available to the recipients for future pregnancies.

- Embryo disposition. The contract should address the intended parents' plans for the disposition of cryopreserved embryos. Since many intended parents may not be able to predict their feelings in the future, all options available to them should be listed as possibilities: donation to another couple (if the egg donor has consented to this), degeneration or donation for scientific research.

- Privacy and communication. Issues of privacy and how information about the egg donation will be communicated, to whom and under what circumstances should be addressed. If future contact is important to you, this must be addressed in your egg donation contract. In addition, it is important that your donor's information continues to be stored by someone so you will have access to this later on if needed.

- Costs. The contract should identify the costs involved in egg donation, including the fee provided to the donor, as well as any costs for medical insurance for the donor and of embryo cryopreservation and storage. In addition, the contract should clearly address who will be responsible for these costs. In almost all cases, the recipient is completely responsible for all costs associated with the egg donation process, including those pertaining to the donor.

- Donor Sibling Registry. Increasing numbers of donors and recipients are writing participation in the Donor Sibling Registry into their contract. The understanding is generally that, if a child is born, both parties will register with the

DSR and remain active in the registry so that medical and other information can be exchanged.

While having a legal contract in place is imperative for anyone pursuing egg donation, it is also important to have realistic expectations, especially regarding issues that might come up after the donation is completed. Even though your donor may have made promises to you in the contract, this does not mean she can be compelled to fulfill these promises. She can breach the contract, giving you the legal right to sue her, but you cannot force her to follow through as planned. Fortunately, you, your physician, your donor egg coordinator, your attorney and your donor's attorney should work together to ensure a successful and positive experience for all and minimize any risk of problems. But, as with everyone, things may change for your donor, causing her to reconsider her promises to you later. While this does not occur often, it is important to be aware of this.

Informed consent

In addition to a legal contract, informed consent must be a goal of egg donation. Informed consent refers to the process that gives patients information about a particular treatment or test so that they can best decide whether or not they should undergo the procedure. The goal is for the patient to understand the risks and benefits involved. Informed consent is based on the moral and legal premise of patient autonomy—the patient has the right to make decisions about his or her own health. Since donating eggs is elective and should be entirely voluntary, informed consent is especially important.

There are four basic components of informed consent:

1. The patient must have the capacity and ability to make the decision.

2. The medical providers must disclose information about the procedure in question, including the expected benefits

and risks, and the likelihood that the benefits and risks will occur.

3. The patient must comprehend the relevant information.

4. Informed consent must be granted voluntarily without any coercion or duress.

The informed consent form must be signed and dated by both the doctor and patient. The patient should always receive a copy of the informed consent as well as have their questions answered about the planned procedure at any time.

Specific legal issues

In the United States, marriage, divorce, child custody and adoption have traditionally been the domain of individual states, all of which have statutes regulating each of these areas. While 30 states have their own laws regarding sperm donation, only a few states (e.g. Florida, North Dakota, Oklahoma, Texas, Washington and Virginia) have laws concerning egg donation. In the United States, there are no statutes preventing people from participating in egg donation and embryo placement, but there are laws that prohibit and criminalize payment for human organs, tissues or babies. Since states vary in their definitions of organ and tissue and in the activities they permit and restrict, paid egg donation could, in some instances, be deemed illegal. Court rulings in adoption, surrogacy and sperm donor cases may also have relevance to egg donation. Internationally, egg donation is governed by a variety of laws, ranging from those in Italy, which bans all forms of egg donation, to those in United Kingdom, which prohibits payment to egg donors. Laws in the United States and worldwide applying to egg donation and other areas of human reproduction are ever-unfolding, and lawyers with practices in reproductive law must pay keen attention to them.

Some common legal concerns expressed by families considering egg donation include the following.

WHO IS THE LEGAL MOTHER? WILL MY CUSTODY OF THE CHILD EVER BE CHALLENGED?

If you give birth to a child, you are considered the legal mother in all cases. For example, being a mother to a child conceived via egg donation cannot be held against you at any time, including custody disagreements or divorce.

Attorney Susan Crockin reports that in a New York case, *MacDonald v. MacDonald*, (*MacDonald v. MacDonald*, 1996 AD2d 7, 608 NYS2d 477 [1994]) a husband attempted to gain custody of twins because he was "the only genetic and natural parent available to them" (Crockin and Jones 2009, pp.188–196). His claim was rejected because the court found "that the couple's intention to jointly have and rear offspring made the recipient woman the 'natural mother of the children'" (ibid). She was granted temporary custody. In the second case of an Ohio couple, *Ezzone v. Ezzone*, a divorcing father claimed that since his wife's sister donated the eggs, she was not the natural mother of her children. The court ruled against the husband, "analogizing his situation to sperm donation and finding an even stronger connection for a woman because she gestates the donated gamete" (ibid). Crockin goes on to say that the court concluded that to treat a woman differently to a man who used donor gametes "would violate both state and federal equal protection laws" (ibid).

Two cases in the UK involved lesbian couples and addressed issues of the rights of non-genetic parents.

The first case was that of *Re v. G* ([2006] UKHL 43(1)) which involved a dispute about where the children conceived to a lesbian couple through artificial insemination should live following the couple's separation. The High Court and Court of Appeal ruled that the non-birth mother should have primary care of the two children (mainly because the birth mother had behaved badly and removed the children to Cornwall deliberately to obstruct her former partner's relationship with the children).

However, in a landmark judgment, the House of Lords ruled that the lower courts had not given sufficient weight to the fact that the birth mother was the biological mother of the children and ordered that the children should continue to live with her. The House of Lords expressly stated that the lower courts had placed too much weight on the behavior of the birth mother and not enough on the biological basis of her relationship. Being the birth mother is, it seems, significant.

The more recent case of *T v. B* ([2010] EWHC 1444 (Fam) (2)) involved a lesbian couple who were not civil partners but had lived together for many years and had undergone fertility treatment to conceive a child together. Once the child was born, they both undertook the role of parents. Although the law at the time did not recognize the non-birth mother as a legal parent, she sought—and was given by the court—parental responsibility, which meant she had full legal authority to take decisions as a parent and to be involved in her child's care.

Following separation, the birth mother applied to the courts for financial provision from the non-birth mother. The court ruled that as the non-birth mother was not a legal parent, she had no financial obligation, despite the fact that she had, to all intents and purposes, been a "parent" from the very start. The court was somewhat constrained by the wording of the law (and its frustration was evident), but it was clear in this case that whether you were a birth mother or not was deeply significant.

On April 6, 2009, the law in the UK changed to allow two mothers to be named on the birth certificate, recognizing them both as the legal parents and giving them both financial responsibility for their children. Both of the UK cases above involved children born before this legal change.

Whether or not the new law will give greater weight to the non-birth mother's position remains to be seen. Things are likely to be muddied further by the increasing blurring of the lines between birth and biological parenthood for lesbian couples. We are certainly seeing more egg-swapping cases, where an egg has been taken from the non-birth mother, fertilized and then transferred to the birth mother. Where parents in these situations separate, will the courts favor the woman who gives birth to the child or the one who provides the egg?

For families who use a gestational carrier and an egg donor, it is important to clarify the laws in the state where the gestational carrier gave birth. Some states require that one or both parents be genetically related to the child in order to circumvent the adoption process all together. In any case, it is critical that you seek the advice of a reproductive attorney in order to work this out well before the birth.

On June 12, 2004, *New York Times* writer Leslie Eaton told the bizarre story of Zack Hampton Bacon III, 51, and Diandra Douglas, 48, an unmarried couple who sought to have children through a gestational carrier and egg donor. The surrogate became pregnant with twin boys and the couple, who had been together since 2000, split up after Ms. Douglas refused to marry Mr. Bacon unless he would pay her the hundreds of thousands of dollars she would lose in alimony from her ex-husband. In addition, Ms. Douglas "was unhappy that the babies were both boys, according to Mr. Bacon's court papers," and, just prior to the twins' birth, "she announced she was planning to adopt a baby girl from Kazakhstan." When the twins were born three months premature, the couple entered into a coast-to-coast custody battle, with Ms. Douglas arguing to be able to raise the boys in California and Mr. Bacon in New York. The fact that Ms. Douglas is not the biological or genetic mother of the twins is unlikely to make a difference legally. The article quotes Attorney Leslie Ellen Shear of Encina, who says that California law emphasizes *intent* when deciding who is a legal parent (Eaton 2004).

CAN A DONOR GAIN PARENTAL RIGHTS?

Prior to July 7, 2004, there was no case on record of an egg donor seeking custody of a child or children created from her eggs. However, in the "brave new world," the following was reported in the *Pittsburgh Post-Gazette* (Stack 2004). A 62-year-old man, James Flynn of Cleveland, Ohio, and his 60-year-old fiancée, Eileen Donich, sought parenthood through an egg donor and a gestational carrier. Following the birth of triplets, the gestational carrier, Danielle Bimber, and the egg donor, identified as "J.R.," both sought custody of the children. Bimber argued that she was the one who had provided the most care for the children, gestating and delivering them, and then, when Flynn failed to produce legal documents to secure custody, Bimber cared for the infants for eight months. Meanwhile, "J.R."—the egg donor, who is reportedly a college student—filed for custody. According to Attorney Steve Litz, the director of Surrogate Mothers, Inc., "J.R." is involved in a scam with Flynn. Litz claims that "J.R." does not want to raise the children, but is cooperating with Flynn.

Aside from this case, which illustrates, in so many ways, the grave need for stricter guidelines in egg donation, there have been no reported cases in which an egg donor, either known or anonymous, has sought parental rights or responsibilities following egg donation. States with statutes regarding egg donation all relieve the egg donor of all parental rights and responsibilities and specifically transfer them to the intended mother.

Attorney Crockin advises looking to the history of sperm donation for further guidance and to predict legal developments in this area. Although the statutes in the states that have regulated sperm donation vary in many ways, all presume that a child born to a married couple is the child of that couple. According to Ms. Crockin, "These laws should, in most states and situations, protect a child and its presumed parents from a sperm donor later attempting to assert parental rights to a child born from his genetic material" (Crockin and Jones 2009, pp.188–196). However, Crockin goes on to say that there have been no reported cases of a previously anonymous sperm donor asserting parental rights and "only a few cases in which a known sperm donor has challenged his status and asserted a claim for paternity" (ibid). In fact, the many lawsuits that have involved children born through sperm donation have involved efforts on the part of the legal father to avoid child support. Crockin notes that these have been uniformly rejected by the courts.

In May 2004, an appeals court in Seattle (Martin 2004) ruled that a sperm donor did not have any rights and responsibilities of fatherhood when he did not sign a consent as required by that state. The case involved Michael Kepl, a man who agreed to give his long-term girlfriend, Teresa Brock, a sperm donation through a University of Washington fertility clinic. Kepl was married and shielded the affair from his wife. Brock gave birth to a son in 1998 and Kepl paid monthly unofficial child support, took out a life insurance policy benefiting the baby and signed a sworn statement of paternity. But the couple did not sign a legally recognized consent form stating that Kepl accepted legal responsibility for the child. The affair crumbled in 2001; Brock went on to have a second child with Kepl's sperm and the two ended up in court. The trial court focused on the consensual nature of the affair and dismissed Kepl's argument that he was only a sperm donor and that Washington state law shields sperm donors from the legal duty of fatherhood, except when couples sign a specific agreement at the time of insemination. However, the appeals court reversed the trial court decision and said that sperm donors can't be forced to accept the rights and responsibilities of parenthood without complying with the statute.

The case may be very significant because it can shield women from donors who later want to intervene in their child's life and it protects sperm (and presumably egg) donors. Lisa Stone, executive director of the Northwest Women's Law Center, suggests if you provide sperm, you're not the father unless there's a separate piece of paper that says this person will be the father and donor (Stone 2004).

The well-known California case of *Johnson v. Calvert* (19 Cal Rptr2d 494 [5.Cal 4th 84] 1993), in which a gestational carrier sought recognition as the mother of a child she carried for a couple, sheds light on the ways that courts might respond to an egg donor attempting to claim parental rights. The California Supreme Court ruled that the natural mother is the one who intended to procreate and raise the child as her own. This reasoning—one that focuses on the intention to parent rather than on genetics—may extend to egg donor situations as well.

Although it is highly unlikely that a donor would ever seek parental rights, let alone be granted them, it is important that the legal contract with your donor clearly states your intent to parent the child that results from egg donation and the donor's clear intent never to seek parental rights.

How are donors legally protected?

The donor needs to be protected in many ways as well. It needs to be made clear precisely when she is donating her eggs and to whom. Even with anonymous donation, you can be designated as the sole recipients of her donation. She has a right to be reassured that you will not pass her eggs on to another couple, either in the form of eggs or as embryos. You will want to know that your donor is also protected financially should she have complications from the procedure that require additional medical treatment.

Just as you need to know that your donor will have no parental rights, so also does she need to know that she will never be held liable for child support or any other maternal obligations to a child born through egg donation. Attorneys recommend that recipient couples agree in writing not to seek such support and to indemnify a donor if the state were to seek such support. In addition, donors and recipients can specifically name their beneficiaries in their wills to avoid any unintended inclusion or exclusion of a child.

What happens if the donor cancels the cycle or does not follow the doctor's instructions?

This is a major reason why it is so important that all donors be carefully screened beforehand. Not only should they be aware of what to expect, but they should understand their responsibilities in this process before the egg donation cycle is even started. It is also critical that the medical program maintains good communication with the donor throughout the cycle so that she feels comfortable asking any questions or letting the clinic know of any problems. Cycles can be postponed or rescheduled for many reasons, and recipient families should anticipate and respect this. While informed consent allows for anyone undergoing any treatment to change her mind at any time, recipient families should have worked very carefully with their reproductive attorney to determine in detail how this will be handled.

WHAT HAPPENS IF THE MEDICAL PROGRAM MAKES A MISTAKE, SUCH AS TRANSFERRING THE WRONG EMBRYOS OR GIVING EGGS TO THE WRONG RECIPIENT?

While still rare, several physicians have been accused of mishandling gametes and embryos in their care. Most recently, the Morell and Savage families found out they were the unexpected victims of an embryo mix-up which Shannon and Paul Morell describe in their book *Misconception: One Couple's Journey from Embryo Mix-Up to Miracle Baby* (2011). In an act of generosity and faith, the Savages handed back baby Logan to the Morells after the birth. The Savages, after years of struggling with infertility and being told that they would not be able to have any more children after this pregnancy, went on to become pregnant with twins via a surrogate a few years later. Logan continues to be healthy and happy, and both families report maintaining a good relationship.

Unfortunately, there are occasional instances when medical and lab errors are not resolved so collaboratively. In one well-publicized instance, physicians at the University of California at Irvine were accused of having mishandled hundreds of gametes, creating embryos without the knowledge or consent of the gamete providers (*Stone v. Regents of Univ. of Cal.* 77 Cal. App. 4th 736, 92 Cal. Rptr. 2nd 94 [1999]). According to Attorney Crockin, the University agreed to pay claimants nearly $17 million to settle claims and at least six children were reportedly born to couples from "erroneously-created or and mis-transferred embryos, using gametes from patients who allegedly never consented to their 'donation' to another couple" (Crockin and Jones 2009, pp.188–196).

Another embryo mix-up occurred in the twin pregnancy of Donna Fasano, who learned that a vial of embryos from the Rogers family had been transferred to her along with her own embryos. The amniocentesis revealed that one of the fetuses was genetically related to the Fasanos, but the other was the Rogers' biological child. The Fasanos initially attempted to parent both children. Following birth, the Rogers' filed suit and successfully obtained legal and physical custody of that child (*Perry-Rogers v. Fasano*, 276 A.D. 2d 67 [NY 2000]). In addition, each family sued their doctors and the laboratory for mixing the embryos (*Fasano v. Nash*, 723. N.Y. S 2d. 181 [App. Div. 2001]) and additional suits for negligence and medical malpractice. In addition to illustrating the legal responsibility that medical programs and their laboratories have to ensure that their patients receive only those gametes and embryos that are theirs, either through biology or donation, this case is also significant for the fact that the court overturned the common law presumption of maternity for Ms. Fasano and gave custody to the genetic parents. It illustrates how critical it is that intent be clear in gamete donation so that no donor can ever claim to have donated "unintentionally."

Again, we hope that you and your medical providers will always be on the same side of the law. These cases of clinic mistakes and of disappointed parents are included not as cautionary tales but rather to illustrate just how careful medical and donor egg programs must be. When you are asked to sign lengthy and complex consent forms, you will have some idea how and why they came to be and why it is so important that you enter egg donation with eyes wide open.

WHAT IF MY CHILD IS BORN WITH A GENETIC DEFECT?

Anyone undertaking pregnancy—with your own eggs or a donor's—knows that a child can be born with a problem or disability. Many disabilities cannot be predicted or avoided. However, there are some genetic issues that can be identified prior to pregnancy and it is these that you trust physicians to screen for prior to attempting pregnancy.

In 2003, a child was born via egg donation with cystic fibrosis. The parents of the child sued for medical malpractice, alleging failure to properly screen the donor, inform the intended parents of the positive screen or test the intended father. New York court dismissed all but one claim which involved the egg donor program's failure to advise parents that their egg donor had been tested and found to be a carrier for cystic fibrosis.

Another widely publicized case involved a sperm bank that allegedly failed to inform recipient couples that a donor had disclosed a family history of kidney disease (*Johnson v. Sup. Ct. of LA*, 101 Cal. App 4th 869 [2002]). A family whose child through sperm donation had kidney disease brought suit against the sperm bank and their physicians. The California appellate court found in favor of the sperm bank and physicians, stating they did not cause the child's genetic abnormality. Similarly, the Utah Supreme Court rejected a case in which a couple who had healthy triplets sued the sperm bank for "negligent infliction of emotional distress" by inseminating the wife with the wrong donor sperm. The parents alleged that they selected a particular donor based on his blood type and hair color, but after birth the children were found to have a different blood type and physical appearance.

Overall, courts have tended to support the complexity of genetics as well as the intended parents' critical role in the health of the child, both genetically and gestationally. A child's health or development is not solely dependent on the egg donor. Moreover, the health of any child cannot be guaranteed by anyone. Thus, parents always take a risk on the outcome of a pregnancy, egg donation or not. Children born via egg donation should not be held to different expectations than any other children born.

What happens if my partner dies?

Given all that you have been through, it is unimaginable that you could be in a donor cycle or pregnant and lose your partner. Still, it is your lawyer's responsibility to cover all possibilities and so the question of what happens to eggs and embryos if an intended parent dies must be addressed. According to the ASRM's policy on Posthumous Reproduction, "If an individual designates the use of stored frozen gametes or embryos that can be used for posthumous pregnancy, either for the use of a spouse or as a donation to others, it would seem to be totally appropriate to honor this designation after that individual's death in the absence of any adverse consequences to the living participants in the pregnancy or any expected children. The gestating woman and/or the rearing parent(s) must be fully informed and in agreement with the process."

Many programs for assisted reproduction have consent forms that stipulate the storage and disposition of gametes and embryos, including disposition after death of one or both gamete donors or after a certain period of time. If the use of the embryos after death is declined, this should be honored. Whether a time limit should be put on how long after death such gametes or embryos might still be used is problematic. It is not clear how the interval between death and use would affect the process and the outcome, but the general presumption is that such use should occur within a few years.

Programs are urged to insist that donors make their wishes known. If no decision on disposition after death has been made, one would expect that in most instances this would preclude any posthumous use.

Legal reform

Each year, laws around egg donation continue to change and evolve in the United States and throughout the world. The main concerns involve issues related to payment and anonymity. Overall, donor compensation "should be fair and not so substantial that they become undue inducements that will lead the donors to discount risks" (ASRM 2007, p.308). While ASRM sets guidelines about appropriate donor payment of between $5000 and $10,000, no specific laws exist in the US. Several countries have banned compensation all together.

Similarly, several states have begun to explore eliminating anonymous egg donors. Washington state passed a law in 2011 guaranteeing children conceived with gametes from Washington egg donation agencies access (when they turn 18) to their donors' medical histories and their full names, unless the donors specifically opt out of being identified.

Some patients and physicians are concerned that there will be state laws created in the future that will be in direct disagreement with contracts drawn up now. Attorney Mark Johnson explains that there are generally proscriptions against retroactive or ex post facto applications of law. In other words, the legal agreements you draw up now will most likely stand the test of time regardless of future changes in the law.

Advocating insurance coverage

In the US, a relatively small number of states have laws mandating insurance coverage for fertility treatment. The specific treatments that insurance companies are required to cover also vary widely from state to state. In most instances, insurance companies are authorized to adopt reasonable guidelines to define what will be covered and what will be excluded. Accordingly, coverage for particular procedures can vary substantially from company to company and some intended parents turn to lawyer's advocates with their insurance plans.

Many insurance companies have used FSH and age (usually somewhere between 40 and 42) to determine whether there should be coverage. Every insurance company has detailed guidelines as to where they will draw the line. If you do not meet these guidelines, you will most likely be denied. Once denied, you have the right to appeal to a review board within the insurance company to overturn the decision. If you are not successful at that level, most policies provide for an external review through either a state agency or an independent review agency under federal law. A lawyer, working in conjunction with your physician, may be helpful with your appeal.

Even in states with mandates, there are insurance carriers that do not offer coverage for fertility treatment. Under the federal Employee Retirement Income Security Act of 1974 (ERISA), self-insured health plans are exempt from state regulation. In addition, state law may also exempt certain employers based on size or some other feature.

Attorney Susan Crockin comments that the Americans with Disabilities Act (ADA), the Civil Rights Act of 1964 and the Pregnancy Discrimination Act of 1978 may all offer patients some potential federal statutory protection in their quest for parenthood (Crockin and Jones 2009). Crockin adds that in the 1998 case, *Bragdon v. Abbott*, the US Supreme Court held "that reproduction constitutes a major life activity under the ADA" (*Bragdon v. Abbott*, 524. U.S. 624, 118 S. Ct. 2196 [1998]). This case involved an HIV positive woman who alleged discrimination in the denial of dental care. The Court reportedly found HIV to be a "disability" that substantially limited a major life activity: reproduction. Crockin observes that even though this decision did not directly involve infertility or insurance coverage, "it may be argued to apply in the context of employer-sponsored health insurance discrimination against those with infertility" (Crockin and Jones 2009, pp.188–196).

Crockin adds that people denied access to infertility treatment can also seek protection under Title VII of the Civil Rights Act of 1964 and the Pregnancy Discrimination Act. The Civil Rights Act prohibits "employment practices that discriminate against an individual with respect to his compensation, terms, conditions, or privileges of employment because of such individual's race, color, religion, sex or national origin" (*Saks v. Franklin Covey Co.* 3`5 F 3d 337 [2nd Cir. 2003]). This prohibition includes discrimination in providing health insurance and benefits. Crockin explains that the Civil Rights Act was amended by the Pregnancy Discrimination Act (PDA) in 1978, an act that forbids discrimination based on "pregnancy, childbirth or related medical conditions." However, she adds that some courts have included infertility in the protections of the PDA and others have not.

For more information about infertility, egg donation and insurance, visit the National Infertility Association at www.resolve.org.

And so we see that egg donation presents a range of psychological challenges and legal puzzles. Because this remains a new frontier, so unique and constantly changing, it is important that you find a mental health counselor and a lawyer who devote their practices to assisted reproduction. They need to be able to provide you with expert guidance during some of the key parts of your journey to parenthood through egg donation.

– 6 –

Attempting Pregnancy
A Collaborative Effort

Egg donation, as you are keenly aware, involves three people working together to create a baby. We turn our attention now to what you can expect when you undergo an egg donation cycle. But since you are not the only patient in this situation, we will focus also on what your husband/partner's role is and on what your donor—whether known or not—will be going through. Protocols and procedures vary worldwide, but here are some of the basics.

Choosing a fertility clinic and assembling the medical team

Many people considering egg donation are already connected to a physician and fertility clinic that they like and trust. If you are among this group, your selection of a medical program is already in place. However, if you are among those individuals or couples who come to egg donation without a history of fertility treatment, or if you have relocated or want, for whatever reason, to find a new program, there are decisions to make. You will want to ask your clinic about their success with egg donation. How many ED cycles do they do each year? What are the ongoing and live delivery rates and what percentage of these pregnancies are multiples? In assessing this information, pay attention to whether there have been any major changes in the program that could improve or diminish the program's success such as the arrival of a new embryologist or changes in the physician staffing.

In the United States, most quality programs are members of ASRM and participate in SART (Society for Assisted Reproductive Technology) and adhere to its reporting and staffing regulations. In addition, all programs using donated eggs (and sperm and embryos) are now required to register with the Food and Drug Administration (FDA). The FDA's regulations—"Eligibility Determination for Donors of Human Cells, Tissues, and Cellular and Tissue-Based Products"—include the regulations that all clinics must adhere to for screening potential donors for infectious diseases, criteria for donor eligibility, specifics about quarantine and storage of reproductive cells, specifics about maintenance of records and the establishment of standard operating procedures.

Since there is no standardized reporting of egg donation success rates to which you can refer, you want to ask the clinic about their pregnancy rates as well as actual birth and multiple birth rates as a result of egg donation. Remember that all this data is self-reported by the fertility clinic, and it is in their best interest to show strong success rates. As a result, all statistical information will have to be taken with a grain of salt. Despite these weaknesses, assessing any egg donor program's statistics should give you some indication about how experienced the clinic is with the procedure and will provide you with opportunities to ask additional questions and get to know the clinic better.

You will also need to find a clinic with which you feel comfortable. You are making a big commitment, not only financially and emotionally but in time and energy. You will want to feel confident that your communication with staff will go well. You need to feel free to ask questions and voice concerns. This may mean interviewing several clinics or physicians to get a better understanding of their backgrounds, their style and the way the staff works together and with clients before making your decision.

The clinic you choose should also have a mental health professional on staff or should be able to refer to a list of qualified counselors who specialize in working with couples struggling with infertility. As we have stressed before, the egg donation process brings with it many emotional and psychological issues, many of which should not be dealt with alone. A good counselor can help guide you through these difficult situations and assist you in making important decisions about the long-term impact of your egg donation.

Remember that egg donation is an intensive process. Your donor must take powerful fertility medications and your cycle must be synchronized with hers. You will want a medical team that is attentive to your donor and to you at all times. They will need to monitor each of you carefully to avoid complications and to increase your chances of becoming pregnant. Since issues can arise at any time during an egg donation cycle, your clinic should have staff available to return phone calls or emails during evenings, weekends and holidays.

Costs

The costs associated with egg donation vary widely depending on where you live, where you might be traveling to, whether you live in a country that permits payment to donors, whether you have chosen a known donor, whether you are using an egg bank and more. Because of these wide variations, we cannot accurately estimate your costs. They may be as little as a few thousand US dollars in some countries and as much as $35,000 in the US. What is important is that you have a handle on costs before you embark upon the process so that you do not encounter surprises or find that you have depleted your savings along the way. Medical programs offering egg donation have financial departments with people who should be well equipped to review all costs with you. Do not be reluctant to ask questions and make sure that you really understand what you will be charged for and when.

If you are working with an agency that recruits donors, be sure to find out what happens if your donor falls through for any reason. Will you be locked in to finding another donor through that agency or will the agency refund all or part of your program fees, freeing you up to look for a donor with another agency?

After you have gathered all of your information about the costs of egg donation and know how much you will be responsible for, you should sit down and plan a budget. How much can you really afford to spend on this particular option to have a baby? Keep in mind that, once you start, it is very easy to get caught up in all the reproductive technologies that are available that might allow you to become pregnant. After all, you may say to yourself, after some unproductive cycles, you just spent $50,000—what's another $10,000 or $20,000? What types of changes and sacrifices will you have to make in your life and lifestyle in order to attempt egg donation? What will you do if egg donation does not work?

As with any major financial decision, it is not uncommon for couples to seek out professional financial advice as to how to organize their money. Egg donation is not just a difficult emotional journey; it can also have a long-lasting financial impact, so we encourage you to make educated decisions in order to protect your future.

Donor testing and screening

Before the egg donation process can be started, the donor must undergo extensive testing and screening to determine if she is an appropriate donor. Whether she is a program-recruited donor or a family member or friend, she will be asked to complete an extensive individual and family medical history questionnaire. This will be followed by medical exams that will focus on both her reproductive and her general health. Physicians will pay particular attention to her menstrual cycle and hormone levels, especially FSH. They will follow FDA regulations which state that egg donors must be tested for infectious diseases up to 30 days before the retrieval. Required blood tests are for HIV-1, HIV-2, hepatitis B and C, syphilis, gonorrhea and chlamydia.

In addition, your donor's genetic history will be evaluated. The American College of Obstetricians and Gynecologists recommends testing for cystic fibrosis, spinal muscular atrophy, Tay-Sachs disease, Canavan disease, familial dysautonomia, Gaucher disease, Fanconi anemia type C, mucolipidosis IV, Bloom syndrome, Niemann-Pick disease type A, beta-thalassemia sickle cell disease, ABCC8-related hyperinsulinism, glycogen storage disease type 1a, maple syrup urine disease type 1b and 3, Usher syndrome, hexosaminidase A deficiency, familial Mediterranean fever, nemaline myopathy and Joubert syndrome. Additional testing that may be completed according to ethnicity: Hb profile (Asian, Mediterranean) or CBC/MCV for alpha-thalassemia (Asian).

Your donor will need to report personal or family history of conditions such as high blood pressure, heart disease, deafness, blindness, severe arthritis, diabetes, alcoholism, schizophrenia, manic depression, epilepsy, Alzheimer's disease, cleft lip or palate, heart defects, clubfoot, spina bifida, color blindness, cystic fibrosis, hemophilia, muscular dystrophy, sickle cell anemia, Huntington's disease, polycystic kidney disease, glaucoma and Tay-Sachs disease.

In addition to genetic problems, your physician will want to confirm that your donor is not significantly overweight, does not smoke and does not have a history of mental illness or a first-degree relative with a history of mental illness. The program mental health counselor may reject her because of a variety of psychological issues, including the recent break-up of a relationship, the death of a loved one and, possibly, a history of sexual abuse.

Intended parents' medical evaluation

In most instances, couples have already endured numerous fertility tests, medications and procedures before approaching egg donation. However, others of you may be new to ART—you may come to egg donation having known for a long time that donor eggs were needed. For this last group, the lingo of ART and the medical procedures will be unfamiliar.

Regardless of where you are in your infertility journey, however, before beginning an egg donation cycle, you will undergo extensive testing to confirm that you are in good health, that your uterus is prepared to accept an embryo and grow a baby, that you are unlikely to have a problem carrying a baby (twins are more challenging) to term. If you haven't already done so, a test will be performed to confirm that the uterine cavity is normal. This can be accomplished by a hysterosalpingogram, sono-hysterogram or hysteroscopy. Especially if you are in your 40s, additional testing, such as mammogram, glucose tolerance test and an electrocardiogram, will probably be requested. In addition, recipients might also be asked to complete basic pre-conception testing such as Pap test, blood count, kidney and liver function, rubella screening, blood Rh factor and thyroid function, in addition to tests for HIV, hepatitis, syphilis, gonorrhea and chlamydia.

Meanwhile, your husband or partner should also complete another semen analysis to ensure that his sperm will be able to fertilize the donor's eggs, as well as having tests for HIV, hepatitis and sexually transmitted infections to avoid spreading these diseases.

In order to ensure your best chances of success, you, your partner and your donor will be instructed to notify the clinic if there are any changes to your health or any medications that are being taken and to avoid smoking, alcohol, caffeine, weight loss programs, vigorous exercise, hot tubs and saunas before and during the egg donation process.

What you can do to prepare physically

As you approach your egg donation cycle, you will probably be wondering what control you have—if any—over its outcome. While there is nothing you can do to ensure that you will have good embryos to transfer, there are ways you can prepare for pregnancy.

"Preparing for pregnancy" may sound like a strange notion, especially if you have never been pregnant. But that is, indeed, what you are doing when you enter into an egg donor cycle—you are taking your first step towards pregnancy. What are some of the steps you can take?

Folic acid and other nutrients

Adequate intake of folic acid has been found to be an essential ingredient of a healthy pregnancy. Many obstetricians now advise that women begin taking folic acid supplements even before a pregnancy test is confirmed. Why not begin taking a prenatal vitamin prior to embryo transfer? Doing so may help create an optimal environment for a fetus.

Diet and nutrition

Along with vitamins and folic acid, you will want to maintain a healthy diet during pregnancy. This is crucial not only for your hoped-for baby's health but also for your own. This may feel especially important to you if you are an older expectant mother and are approaching egg donation with concerns about your age. A diet rich in fruits, brightly colored vegetables, protein and calcium can assist you in maintaining your general health.

There are some reports that bromelain, found in pineapples, helps implantation. Others credit walnuts with launching a pregnancy. In both instances, reports are largely anecdotal, but unless you are allergic to walnuts or pineapple, we see no reason why you shouldn't include them in your pre-transfer and during transfer diet. Both are known to be health-promoting foods and eating them may help you feel that you are doing all you can to make a home for the embryo.

Exercise

"Exercise—it's good for you and reduces stress." "Don't exercise when you are in the midst of a cycle." You are probably confused by the conflicting advice you receive about exercise. While most physicians say that it is okay—or even a good idea—to maintain moderate exercise, you should talk specifically with your doctor about what he or she advises for you. The key, we feel, is balance: you will not want to be sitting on the couch and worrying about your cycle, but this is not a good time to begin training for a marathon.

What you can do to prepare emotionally

In addition to preparing physically for pregnancy through egg donation, you should be prepared emotionally as well. It may be helpful to anticipate feeling some—if not all—of the following.

Ambivalence

"Do we really want to do this?"

You thought you were sure. You thought you'd put doubts behind you. Now they creep in again and you wonder what they mean. Does this mean that you don't really want to attempt pregnancy through egg donation? Does this mean you haven't "resolved" your infertility?

Please remember that it is okay to be ambivalent. In fact, it is difficult for us to imagine anyone moving forward without ambivalence. You are making a huge decision: anyone who attempts pregnancy—whether on their own or through donated gametes—is making a lifelong commitment to a total stranger. How scary is that? When you think of it that way, can you imagine someone feeling 100 percent convinced that they are doing the right thing?

Fear that it won't work

"Egg donation has great success rates." That's what you have been hearing for a long time. Now that you are about to begin a cycle, you wonder, "But what if it doesn't work? What will this mean about me if I can't even become pregnant with a donated egg?" Egg donation does not always work, and, when it doesn't, women tend to feel very responsible and very much to blame. They are also left feeling betrayed by their bodies, which don't seem to work at all—even with "good" eggs.

Women whose sisters or friends are donating to them have additional motivation for wanting a cycle to work. "After all we are putting her through, I will feel terrible if it doesn't work." If this is the situation you are in, try to remember that your sister, cousin or friend is donating because she wants you to have a chance to have a baby. The counseling she has received has amply warned her that her donation in no way guarantees a successful pregnancy.

Fear that you will feel like a fake

You've worked hard to make sense of egg donation and to feel confident that, if it works, you will be a full and legitimate mother. Still there is that old nagging fear that this hoped-for pregnancy won't feel right, that others will somehow identify you as different, that you will feel obliged to tell everyone who notices your growing belly that "it's a donor egg."

We remind you, yet again, that you have a right to privacy and to authenticity. Your child will need to know the truth about his origins and he has the right to tell others his personal story. But, beyond this, you have no obligation to tell anyone how you conceived. Think about it: do your fertile friends tell you their "getting pregnant" stories?

Loss

No one grows up looking forward to having a baby through egg donation. No matter how you got here, there have been losses along the way—failed cycles, pregnancy losses, perhaps the loss of your ovaries due to serious illness. Regardless of how much you may want to do it, egg donation is a second choice.

Looking around you at other women going through egg donation, you are likely to notice different reactions to loss. Those of you who were older when you married or began to attempt pregnancy probably spent many years fearing that you would never have a child. For you, the opportunity for pregnancy through egg donation may feel more like a miracle or a gift than a loss. Your journey has been decidedly different from fellow travelers who may have experienced premature ovarian failure and arrived at the choice to use donated egg somewhat shell-shocked by what has happened to them. There are also those in their late 30s or early 40s who come to egg donation only after years of fertility treatment, failed cycles or pregnancy losses. And there are single women who had hoped to be doing this with a partner.

Regardless of what brought you to egg donation, loss is part of your experience. As you move forward, loss will travel with you. We hope that your donor cycle will lead to the joyous arrival of a baby you will love and cherish. Still, this will not be your genetic child.

> Nancy, 37, who is eight months pregnant through egg donation, put it this way: "This baby is our dream come true, and yet I still feel that someone has died."

Your feelings of loss will shift as you make your way along your journey. The woman who spoke of such profound loss when she was eight months pregnant was giddy with delight when her son was born. Her reaction is a common one: women are relieved and thrilled when they finally give birth to a healthy baby.

Hope and anticipation

It has probably been a long time since you have felt hopeful about pregnancy. You are now at a point where hope is appropriate and anticipation makes sense. Egg donation isn't a sure bet, but it does bring many, many babies into the world. You have reason to hope that yours will be one of them.

Beginning the cycle

Ovarian suppression, stimulation and monitoring

The very first step of the egg donation process is on Day 2 or 3 of the menstrual cycle: both the donor and intended mother have baseline ultrasounds and blood tests. Next, the donor and intended mother will have their cycles synchronized using oral contraceptives and/or Lupron. Oral contraceptives help start the ovarian suppression process and are continued for 2–4 weeks. Lupron is begun about two weeks before the start of the ovarian stimulation and often overlaps with the oral contraceptives. To ensure ovarian suppression is achieved, an ultrasound and blood testing is usually performed.

Once the donor and intended mother have both achieved low estrogen levels, the donor begins daily dosage of injectable fertility medications, while Lupron is continued at a lower dose. These medications are usually self-administered under the skin. The actual fertility drug combination varies, depending on a number of factors such as the patient's age and weight. Also, doctors have their own specific protocol based on their experience, and, depending on your and the donor's reaction to this protocol, changes might have to be made. During this time, the intended mother begins also oral estrogen therapy. Estrogen helps prepare the uterus and uterine lining for embryo transfer.

For the next few days, regular office visits will start for the donor. These continue every 1–2 days until the egg retrieval takes place. Ultrasounds and blood tests for estradiol are performed at each visit. At the end of each day, the donor is called to receive further medication instructions. Based on the donor's monitoring, the intended mother's cycle is adjusted to the donor's cycle.

Additionally, the intended mother will begin taking progesterone before the embryo transfer is scheduled. Again, this helps to mature the lining of the uterus to allow implantation. Progesterone levels are very critical for all pregnant women during early pregnancy in order to maintain the pregnancy. To ensure adequate progesterone levels, most fertility specialists recommend that egg donation recipients continue progesterone supplementation throughout the first trimester of the pregnancy. After the first trimester, the placenta takes over maintaining appropriate hormone levels for the baby. Progesterone should be natural, not synthetic, and is taken most often via intramuscular injection. Unfortunately, these injections are uncomfortable, leaving many newly pregnant women with sore bums. You may be spared this as some programs prescribe progesterone in a vaginal suppository or vaginal gel.

As with all medications, some of the fertility medications may have side effects. This is why it is so important that both donor and recipient are monitored very closely throughout the process. Some side effects that occur in about 10 percent of women can include pelvic pain, nausea and vomiting, hot flashes, bloating, abdominal cramping, mood changes, breast tenderness, blurred vision and rashes or hives. It is vital that recipient or donor call the clinic immediately if either experiences any of these side effects at any point in treatment.

For your donor, some of these side effects may be early warning signs of ovarian hyperstimulation syndrome (OHSS) since her ovaries are being prepared to produce many eggs at the same time. OHSS occurs in about 1–2 percent of donors. It occurs when too many follicles are stimulated, causing the ovary to become enlarged. If left untreated, OHSS can worsen quickly and develop into a serious medical condition. Again, we stress that if a donor experiences any adverse side effects or if she suspects that she could have OHSS, she should call the doctor right away. It is much better to be safe than sorry.

Administering injections

Both you and your egg donor may be giving yourselves injections, sometimes daily, for several weeks. At first it can seem intimidating, but most women become confident with their new skills in a short time.

Your physician or a nurse will explain the medication schedule as timing of the medications is important. Make sure you do not miss a dose or forget to administer the injection. While it is desirable to take the medication at roughly the same time every day, an hour or two earlier or later probably will not make a difference. Make sure you completely understand your medication schedule and do not be afraid to ask questions if you are unsure. Also, make sure you know whom to call if questions arise once you get home.

The first step is to find a clean, quiet and comfortable place to administer the injections. Wash and dry your hands thoroughly. Get all of your supplies together, including the injectable fertility medications, any fluids needed to dilute the drugs, syringes, needles, alcohol swabs and a sharps container to dispose of your used needles. Next, mix the fertility drugs as the directions indicate. Some will need to be diluted, others require mixing and some used straight out of the bottle.

You will need to find a site where you will inject the fertility drugs. Many women find the most convenient and comfortable site to be the belly, although you should try to avoid the area right around the belly button. Clean the area with an alcohol swab and let it dry. Now it is time to inject the drug. Use your non-dominant hand to pinch a fold of skin and hold it. Then use your dominant hand to pick up the syringe and quickly puncture the fold of the skin. Keep the needle there as you slowly push the plunger down. After the plunger is down, rapidly withdraw the needle. Use an alcohol swab to keep pressure on the site for a moment or two.

Finally, you will need to dispose of your sharps appropriately in a special container, clean the area and put away your medications.

If you really don't think you can do it, you might want to recruit a close friend or family member, such as your husband, to give you these injections. The person you choose should feel comfortable with doing this and should also talk to the pharmacist or physician to make sure he or she understands how to handle and prepare the medications.

For more information about injectable fertility medications and video injection lessons, visit Village Fertility Pharmacy (www.villagefertilitypharmacy.com).

Ovulation induction and egg retrieval

Usually, between Days 8–12 when the follicles are large enough, final egg maturation is triggered with an injection of human chorionic gonadotropin (hCG). The timing of the hCG injection is very important as the egg retrieval is performed 36 hours later.

The actual egg retrieval procedure takes about 30 minutes. Depending on the clinic, a light anesthesia or "twilight sleep" is used during the procedure. Additionally, some women experience nausea during this procedure so an anti-nausea medication may also be recommended. A transvaginal ultrasound is inserted into the vagina to help the physician position the ovaries. He or she guides a suctioning needle into the follicle and the fluid is removed. The fluids are then examined by an embryologist who identifies the eggs. Following this egg retrieval process, the donor usually remains in the clinic for 1–2 hours before returning home. Anywhere between five and 35 eggs are typically retrieved. Although greater numbers of eggs generally bode well for ultimate success (since you are likely to have cryopreserved embryos available for future transfer), having fewer eggs does not mean you will not achieve pregnancy.

Egg retrieval—for both donor and recipient—is a stressful time. You will be worrying about what your donor is going through—especially if she is your sister or someone else close to you—and you will be focusing on the outcome of the retrieval. Try to remember that this is a process over which you have no control. Be fair to yourself and don't hold yourself responsible if your donor has an uncomfortable procedure or if only a small quantity of eggs are obtained.

It is important to remember that even though egg retrieval does not involve any incisions, it is surgery. While relatively rare, some donors may suffer damage to organs that are within close proximity to the ovaries. Other complications may include trauma to the ovaries, infection, vaginal bleeding and lacerations. These complications may necessitate a hospitalization and possible surgery. Your egg donor must realize that a consequence of a complication is that it may impact her health or future fertility. Fortunately, serious complications are rare and the vast majority of egg retrievals proceed uneventfully.

Your donor will need to have someone drive her home after the procedure, and she is usually advised to rest for the remainder of the day. Again, if she is someone close to you, it is likely that you will be with her, tending to her discomfort and letting her know how much you appreciate what she has been through. If she is a program-recruited donor with whom you are not in contact, you will surely be thinking of her, perhaps sending her flowers or a small gift. Know that responsible programs will make sure that she is well cared for after retrieval. It is also their job to stay in close contact with her to be sure she is recovering uneventfully, both physically and emotionally.

Sperm samples

Before egg retrieval, your husband or partner will have to provide a sperm sample. The two of you should talk to your fertility specialist about the best time to collect the sample. Fresh sperm obtained on the day of egg retrieval is usually most desirable for fertilizing the egg. However, many couples feel uncomfortable waiting until the last possible minute and risking the chance that the male partner may feel too stressed about the pressure to produce a sperm sample on demand. While not ideal, it is possible that the sperm sample can be provided early and frozen until the eggs are retrieved and ready for fertilization.

In order to increase the chances that a good sperm sample is provided, men are asked to notify the clinic if any illness involving a fever or a sexually transmitted infection has occurred in the last few months. They are also asked to avoid hot tubs, saunas, drugs, alcohol, smoking and vigorous exercise. Men are encouraged to abstain from having intercourse for at least two days before the sample is given.

Fertilization—creating an embryo

Immediately after the egg retrieval, the egg meets up with the sperm. In some cases, intracytoplasmic sperm injection (ICSI) is performed. With ICSI, the sperm is injected directly into the egg by the embryologist to encourage fertilization. Sometimes assisted hatching is used. This is done by creating a small hole in the outer shell of the egg to facilitate hatching and implantation.

However, there is still no guarantee that any of the eggs undergoing these types of micromanipulation will fertilize or implant. For example, with ICSI, there is no way to know for sure which are the best sperm to choose for injection.

The eggs are then checked the next day to determine which ones have fertilized.

Embryo quality and development

Of course, your physician will want to select the best embryos for transfer in order to maximize your chance for pregnancy. Embryos are graded by an embryologist to assess their quality. This grading looks at cell number and fragmentation. Embryo fragmentation refers to the problem of cells of an embryo splitting off into small fragments. This is considered normal and is expected to some extent among all embryos. However, an excessive amount of fragmentation is indicative of a lower-quality embryo. Up to 10 percent fragmentation is considered good quality, 10–20 percent is okay and more than 20 percent is considered suboptimal. While a successful pregnancy can be achieved with a fragmented embryo, the odds decrease as fragmentation increases.

Day 3 embryos are ranked by the number of cells that are present, along with a score from 1, being the best, to 4, being the worst. Alternatively, embryos can be assessed at Day 5 when they are at the blastocyst stage using the ranking AA-quality, considered the best (rarely seen in the laboratory), to DD-quality, those most likely unsuitable for transfer. Deciding how long to let the embryos develop can be a confusing decision. Physicians vary in their opinions about the optimal time for embryo transfer. Some recommend transferring the embryos on Day 3, while others like to wait until the embryo has reached the blastocyst state (Day 5). This is an area of controversy and a real Catch-22 situation. On the one hand, if you transfer the embryos early, you will have more to transfer in the hope that one will make it. On the other hand, if you wait until the embryos have had time to further develop, you might have very few, if any, embryos still available to be transferred. However, each of these embryos will have a higher chance of success than less-developed embryos. Because this is such a difficult decision and there are no definitive answers, you should talk with your physician about his/her perspective. Every clinic has had different experiences with embryo transfers. In any case, this decision should be well informed and made on a case-by-case basis, depending on how your embryos are developing in the laboratory.

Although we hope and expect that you will have had a conversation with your physician at the start of the cycle about how many embryos to transfer, it is possible that there will be additional discussion at this point. Since the goal for all fertility clinics is a singleton pregnancy, with twins but no higher-order multiples being an acceptable outcome, most physicians recommend transferring one or two high-quality embryos. This practice is common because transferring two high-quality embryos usually results in no greater than a twin pregnancy. There have been, however, occasional instances in which an embryo splits. For example, I (Ellen) have an egg donation patient who had two unsuccessful transfers; on the third frozen transfer, two thawed embryos resulted in a triplet pregnancy that included identical twins. You will probably be planning on transferring one or two "high-quality" embryos, but what if you have only three "mediocre" ones? Occasionally, your physician may encourage you to transfer all three, knowing, of course, that you run the risk of a triplet pregnancy. About one in four of all ART pregnancies results in multiple gestation, the majority of which are twins.

PGD and PGS

Preimplantation genetic diagnosis (PGD) and preimplantation genetic screening (PGS) are techniques that provide diagnostic information concerning an embryo before it is transferred to the uterus. PGD and PGS involve removing one or two cells from a six- to eight-cell embryo, usually three days after fertilization. PGD is often used by couples undergoing ART who have significant concerns that a genetic disease may be passed to their child, leading to pregnancy loss or the birth of a severely ill child, such as Fragile X syndrome, Down syndrome, Tay-Sachs disease, Duchenne muscular dystrophy, hemophilia, Turner syndrome,

Huntington's disease and cystic fibrosis. PGS is similar to PGD, but it often includes couples without an underlying genetic problem in order to identify those embryos that are genetically abnormal so that improved embryo selection may result in improved pregnancy rates.

What role do PGD and PGS have in egg donation? Most often, there is little indication for either of these since egg donors are carefully screened for genetic disorders and male partners should be screened as well. However, there will occasionally be situations in which these techniques can be helpful. These are most likely to occur in intrafamily donation—if your sister is your donor and there is a question of some genetic disorder in your family or in your husband's.

Number of embryos

The number of embryos to be transferred is a big decision and one that you should talk about carefully with your doctor as early in the process as possible. Many of us might think "the more the better" or even "two for the price of one," but this is not the case when it comes to embryos. While it is true that not all the embryos transferred will implant into the uterus, you should be prepared to be pregnant with however many embryos you transfer. In fact, ASRM recommends guidelines for appropriate embryo numbers transferred based on age, and many fertility experts advocate for single embryo transfers (SET). While these measures have greatly reduced the incidence of triplets and higher-order multiples, the incidence of twins remains high with egg donation. And multiple births can be problematic for both mother and babies. For example, twins have about a 50 percent chance of being born prematurely, increasing the risk for cerebral palsy and other complications of maturity. Moreover, from conception to delivery, there is a reduced chance of actually delivering two live babies. While twins might seem cute and a bargain at first, families undergoing egg donation should inform themselves about the risks of multiple births and the potential of a single embryo transfer with their physician.

Embryo transfer

Embryo transfer takes place either three or five days after the egg retrieval, depending on the development of the embryo. The embryo transfer is a simple procedure performed by placing a soft catheter containing the embryos through the cervix, using an ultrasound for guidance. Embryo transfers do not require anesthesia, but many women do opt to take Valium to help them relax, mentally and physically with regard to the pelvic muscles. As a result, it is important that women undergoing an embryo transfer arrange for a ride home. Patients are typically asked to arrive 30 minutes before the procedure and must remain lying down for at least 15 minutes following the procedure.

Within a few hours, you will be sent home to wait and wonder, "Did it work?" Once home, you will be advised to rest for the first 24 hours after the embryo transfer and engage in only limited activity. After about 24 hours, you will be told that you can resume normal activities. However, for many women, this is easier said than done. Up until this point you have had virtually no control over the outcome of the cycle. In fact, what you do or don't do probably still has no impact on what happens, but now it feels different. Live embryos have been placed inside you, and you are likely to feel responsible. Your donor did her part. Your husband did his part. Your physician and embryologist did their parts. Now it feels as if it is up to you. Not surprisingly, many hopeful moms avoid exercise, eat well, and rest, hoping to help the embryo find a secure home in their womb.

Try to remember that, as far as anyone knows, there is really nothing you can do to increase your chances of a successful outcome. All depends on the quality of the embryos and the post-transfer hormonal support, neither of which you can control. Therefore, if you can, you should go about your regular daily activities without worrying that you will harm a potential pregnancy. If this is difficult—and we expect it to be—try to remember that staying busy helps distract you a bit and this can help reduce stress. While we are not saying that stress prevents implantation, stress does make the experience more difficult for both you and your partner.

Additional embryos and cryopreservation

One of the benefits of a fertile egg donor is that she is likely to produce several high-quality eggs, which may result in several good-quality embryos. If there are more good-quality embryos than can be safely transferred at one time, there are several options to consider. It is important to think about your decision before you are faced with it. Many counselors bring up this issue during the pre-screening counseling session. All of these options for dealing with extra embryos bring with them important considerations.

Many couples have additional embryos cryopreserved for later use. It is not unusual for a first cycle to fail and for a couple to achieve pregnancy on a frozen or thaw cycle. It is also not unusual for couples to have a child, wait a year or two or three and return to have cryopreserved embryos transferred in the hope of a second pregnancy.

Embryos are frozen in small protective straws at about −40 degrees Celsius in a liquid nitrogen tank. Research has shown that good-quality embryos often freeze well and that there are no significant differences between fresh and cryopreserved embryos when it comes to successful pregnancy rates. It is unclear exactly how long embryos can be cryopreserved. While there remain embryos cryopreserved since the dawn of IVF over 30 years ago, most researchers suggest using embryos that have been cryopreserved for less than five years if possible. Additionally, not all embryos will be suitable for freezing. The embryologist will carefully evaluate the embryos and eliminate the poor-quality embryos that will not be able to survive the freeze and thaw procedures. Many clinics charge couples yearly or monthly storage fees for these cryopreserved embryos. For those couples who cannot afford these ongoing fees, maintaining cryopreserved embryos might not be possible.

But what do you do if you complete your family during your first cycle or decide for some other reason not to use your cryopreserved embryos? Basically, you have three options.

One option is to donate embryos to scientific study, such as stem cell research. This is not always easy to accomplish, but some clinics do have arrangements that facilitate donation to science. In a *Boston Globe* article in 2002, entitled "A worthy gift, a difficult task," I (Ellen) told of Mark and Carla, a couple who worked long and hard to donate their embryos and, who, with the help of Dr. Steven Bayer of Boston-IVF, were able to donate them to a program at Harvard University for Parkinson's disease research. Carla and Mark, devout Catholics, came to this decision because "we wanted to help others but we could not imagine someone else raising our biological children."

Other families choose embryo placement—offering their embryos to another infertile couple. This is a different experience for those whose donor is a family member or friend rather than a program-recruited donor. When a sister or close friend has donated her eggs, our sense is that the embryos may feel more like a personal gift that needs to be kept in the family. In contrast, this option may make sense for egg donor parents who worked with program-recruited donors—the embryos are already partially from someone outside their genetic family, so why not pass them on to someone who needs them? However, this decision brings with it many ethical and some legal issues, including the intent of the donor when she donated her eggs to you. If embryo placement interests you, make sure to discuss this with your reproductive attorney beforehand to ensure it is clearly spelled out in your contract. Many clinics are reluctant to participate in embryo placement without the consent of the donor.

Finally, there is the option of allowing degeneration to occur. Thawed embryos usually degenerate quickly, and continued growth is impossible without placement into the uterus. Most often this is done in a laboratory setting; however, a few women have chosen to place these embryos into their vaginas in order to provide a more natural environment within their bodies for the embryos to degenerate. There is no chance for pregnancy to occur using this method, since the embryos cannot travel from the vagina to the uterus.

For parents who have gone through complicated measures such as egg donation to have a child, it may be difficult to part with their embryos and decide their eventual fate. Cheryl Meyer, author of *The Wandering Uterus*, explains that for some couples the choice may be out of their hands. Some states and countries prohibit the destruction of embryos, and others severely restrict the use of embryos for research. However, for the most part, couples with cryopreserved embryos will eventually be forced to contemplate the fate of their "could-be" children.

Pregnancy testing

Pregnancy tests make it possible to know that you are pregnant less than two weeks following transfer of embryo(s). Pregnancy is determined by detecting hCG level in your urine or blood. While urine pregnancy tests are quick, they can be vague, especially during early pregnancy when the hCG levels are still low. Blood pregnancy tests can determine the exact level of hCG in your body, indicating whether or not you are indeed pregnant. Sometimes, the blood hCG test may be repeated again a few days later since the value should double every 2–3 days in a viable pregnancy.

With egg donation, most doctors recommend having a blood hCG test (often called a Beta test) about 12 days after the embryo transfer. If the hCG levels are low (5 or less), the cycle did not work. Levels in the middle range (5–25) are often inconclusive, so another test will be recommended 48–72 hours later to see if the levels are rising. Higher levels indicate the cycle worked.

Most women find these two weeks between the embryo transfer and pregnancy testing to be excruciating. They try to figure out if they are pregnant by feeling for breast tenderness, wondering if they are unusually fatigued or perhaps a bit nauseous. Unfortunately, it is difficult to make sense of symptoms since you are still taking progesterone, which has side effects that mimic the early symptoms of pregnancy. Once a pregnancy is confirmed, an ultrasound is usually performed 4–5 weeks after the transfer to assess the growing embryo as well as the number of embryos. And so you come to the end of an egg donor cycle.

This ending may also be a new beginning—the beginning of your pregnancy. Or it may represent yet another of the difficult junctures in your journey to parenthood. We hope that those of you who are not pregnant after one cycle will have embryos available for subsequent transfer or that you will feel prepared to travel down a different path. We hope, most of all, that you feel good about the efforts that you and your donor made and satisfied that you can move on without feelings of regret.

– 7 –

Pregnancy with Donated Eggs

You are standing in line at the ATM machine and notice that the woman in front of you is at least seven months pregnant. She looks content and cute in her maternity capri pants and turtleneck. You leave the bank feeling sad and envious. As you are getting into your car, you see a woman walk by, pushing a twin stroller. Seated in front of her are her two little boys—perhaps seven or eight months old—seated upright and apparently enjoying the ride. You drive off convinced there is practically a conspiracy of parents—they are planted everywhere to plague you.

Consider this. The woman at the ATM may be carrying a baby conceived through egg donation. The twins could very likely be donor offspring. Last week when you were in church or synagogue and a baby was baptized or named, did you stop to think that those families too may have been helped along by other women?

We hope our point is clear: you are not alone. If you are newly pregnant through egg donation, CONGRATULATIONS! You have worked hard to get here and, as you can tell from the start of your pregnancy, there is more work to be done. In this chapter, we will begin with some of the feelings you may encounter as your pregnancy unfolds and move on to some of the tasks that lie ahead.

Pregnancy

> I wasn't able to create my baby, but I realized, as soon as I learned I was pregnant, that I would do everything in my power to make sure he had a good start in life. I had taken good care of myself with my pregnancy with my daughter years earlier, but this time I was hyper-vigilant—no caffeine, no vigorous exercise, milk ten times a day, and enough broccoli, carrots and tomatoes to feed an army of vegetarians. (Kathy, 37)

"Taking good care of my baby." These are the watch words of women pregnant with donated eggs. In addition to the caution, appreciation and sense of wonder felt by all infertile expectant moms, egg donation moms-to-be feel an added responsibility: to grow their babies well. Like Kathy, they couldn't create their children, but they can do all they can to take care of them.

Why does it feel so important? Why do women pregnant through egg donation regard eating right and sleeping right and thinking right and moving right to be such a sacred responsibility? It is important to note that these are the feelings of many women pregnant after infertility. However, they may be all the more powerful for you. You may feel that if you couldn't create your child, you want to do all you can to grow him well during pregnancy. So what can you do to help your baby get a good start in life? We turn here to common medical and emotional questions.

The impact of high-tech conception

"You can't be a little bit pregnant." That's what they always told you, but now that you are pregnant through egg donation, you doubt the truth of that old adage. Like other women pregnant after IVF, whether with their own eggs or with donated eggs, you can feel a little bit pregnant from the time you learn there are fertilized embryos in a lab. You are a little bit more pregnant when there is a positive pregnancy test and this little bit increases as the pregnancy hormones rise.

The good news is that women do begin to feel *really pregnant* somewhere along the way. Best we can tell, it is usually around the beginning of the second trimester that women pregnant with donated eggs really begin to think, "Yes, I am pregnant. Yes, there may really be a baby at the end of this journey." Many women report that the pregnancy feels real to them when they feel the baby move.

One of the reasons that the role of technology diminishes as the pregnancy progresses is that pregnant women are referred on from reproductive medicine programs to obstetricians programs at around week 9 or 10. Most who are carrying singletons land in the offices of regular ob-gyns. Difficult as this may be to believe, obstetricians and their staffs regard pregnancy as an entirely natural, commonplace, uneventful experience. While it may be a bit startling to encounter a calm, "nothing to worry about" welcome, this may be the beginning of you feeling like a "normal," pregnant woman. The words "Everything looks fine, take your prenatal vitamins and I will see you in a month" mark a shift from the step-by-step crawl towards pregnancy that you've experienced over the past many months or even years.

Los Angeles Marriage and Family Therapist, Carole Lieber Wilkins, who has worked with many women pregnant after egg donation, observes that many of the women she meets with feel a sense of panic rather than relief when an obstetrician takes an "everything's normal" approach. She reports that some of her patients wish they could have their "own personal ultrasound machine" in order to continue to be closely monitored.

Not everyone is referred to a regular ob-gyn and not everyone's egg donation pregnancy is uneventful. If you find yourself carrying twins, you may decide that you are more comfortable with a high-risk obstetrician, particularly someone affiliated with a hospital that has a level 1 neonatal unit (this is the highest level of infant care and important in multiple gestation when babies come early). If you have diabetes, an incompetent cervix, or any other condition that puts you at risk for complications during your pregnancy, you will probably be encouraged to work with a high-risk obstetrician.

Obstetrical care

You found a good reproductive endocrinologist, you worked well with him (or her) and now you are pregnant. At some point fairly on in your pregnancy—usually around week 8 or 9—you will graduate to an obstetrician. Although congratulations are very much in order, it is not always so easy moving on. Your reproductive endocrinologist may be someone you have been working with for years. He (or she) knows you well, knows how special this pregnancy is, how vulnerable you feel. He is sensitive to privacy issues. It may have been this physician who helped you through a pregnancy loss or with the decision to turn to your sister or a friend or program donor for eggs. But reproductive endocrinologists don't usually offer obstetrical care. It's time to find a doctor who does.

Some of you may be returning to a physician you know well. Your obstetrician may have been your gynecologist for years. He may have delivered your first child, if you have secondary infertility. Or perhaps it was this doctor who did your initial infertility testing. He may be the one who found your reproductive endocrinologist for you.

But for those of you who do not have an obstetrician you want to return to, we have some suggestions for how to choose an obstetrician.

Seek a physician who delivers at a facility in which you have confidence. Childbirth services vary from one hospital to the next and not all medical centers have neonatal intensive care units. In addition, there are different levels of neonatal care, with only a limited number of hospitals offering the highest level. While we hope that you deliver a full-term, healthy baby, it can be reassuring to know that there is the highest level of neonatal intensive care available, should you need it.

You also want to be able to be open, honest and vulnerable with your physician. Obstetricians are busy, and, in the US, medical malpractice cases have made their work stressful. Still, there are many dedicated obstetricians who love what they do and who genuinely enjoy accompanying women through pregnancy.

It will be important for you to find someone who is comfortable with egg donation and who will convey to you a sense that your pregnancy, while very special, is a *regular* pregnancy.

Pay attention to your obstetrician's staffing, especially with regard to coverage. If your obstetrician is a sole practitioner, you will want to know who will cover for him, should you need to call during a vacation or on a weekend. Who will deliver your baby if your doctor is unavailable? If he is in a group practice, you should ask whether you will be seeing different doctors for each visit, and what the chances are that one of them will be delivering your baby.

Look also at the efficiency and lines of communication in the practice. Do you get a machine with several prompts each time you call, or do you get to talk with a real person? This may sound trivial, but if you are bleeding or have some other concern about your pregnancy, you will want to know that you can reach someone and have a prompt response to your concerns.

Talk with your reproductive endocrinologist about whether you should see a high-risk obstetrician, and, if so, whom he recommends. If you are over 45 or carrying multiples, you may well be referred to a high-risk doctor. However, if you are younger, carrying a singleton and have no risks such as diabetes, you are probably headed for a regular obstetrician. This makes sense medically, but does it also make sense emotionally? This pregnancy is very precious to you, and you may benefit from the added attention that comes in a high-risk practice.

Being in the care of a high-risk obstetrician can be a mixed experience for women pregnant through egg donation. On the one hand, it can be comforting and reassuring to feel that you are going to receive that extra measure of care. You don't really feel just like everyone else and so it can be helpful to know that you won't be treated just like everyone else. On the other hand, there is something reassuring about the calm, "there is nothing different about your pregnancy" approach that many women with egg donation pregnancies receive.

Prenatal testing

As with all pregnant women, you will, most likely, be undergoing some prenatal testing regardless of the age of your donor, your husband, genetic family histories and so on. This testing should be reassuring. Ultrasound monitoring is an integral part of contemporary obstetrical care. Ultrasounds will offer you an opportunity to see your baby grow and should help make him more real to you. Blood tests that indicate assorted levels are within normal range should provide you with additional assurance that things are going well.

It is also possible, however, that this routine prenatal testing will prompt concerns. If one of the practitioners caring for you notices something that concerns him or her, additional testing may be suggested. Should this occur, it will be upsetting, but we hope that the outcome will be as it was for my (Ellen) friends. They are both very short people, and their donor, a sister, is quite petite. During the seventh month, a routine ultrasound indicated the baby was "small." After a flurry of tests, the doctors concluded that there was no reason for alarm, at which point the expectant grandfather, himself a pediatrician, said, "I wished they had looked at the height of the parents before worrying that their baby was small."

During your pregnancy some of you will face questions about prenatal testing. Perhaps a concern is raised by an ultrasound or blood test. There may be another reason for testing, such as a genetic disease in the family (this will depend on the nature of the genetic disorder and of the chances that the donor, as well as the expectant father, are carriers) or because the donor (perhaps a sister or friend) is over 35, or because the expectant father is in his late 40s or 50s.

Before deciding to undergo any of the invasive prenatal tests such as chorionic villus sample (CVS) or amniocentesis, you will want to carefully consider why you are having the test. Would you ever terminate a pregnancy? If so, under what conditions? If you would not, is there reason to have the test? Some of you may feel that you would want to know, in advance, that you were expecting a child with a particular condition so that you could feel more prepared. However, you will need to consider whether the added preparation is worth the potential risks involved with prenatal testing. Each procedure carries with it some risk of pregnancy loss, a risk that will vary depending upon the test, the skill of the person performing it and the timing of the test.

Nutrition, exercise and general health

As we noted earlier, you will want to take very good care of yourself during pregnancy. Remember, though, not to go overboard. Women who have gone through years of infertility and those who choose egg donation often make promises along the way. "If I am ever pregnant, I will eat lots of fruits and vegetables." "If I am pregnant, I won't drink or have a lot of caffeine." "If I am pregnant, I will cut back on my running, perhaps shift to walking or swimming." These may all be good ideas, but try not to take them to an extreme. Eating lots of vegetables doesn't mean ten servings of broccoli daily, nor does it mean removing every last French fry from your diet. Staying away from alcohol doesn't mean you can't drink a little champagne at your sister's wedding or enjoy some chicken cooked in wine. And limiting rigorous exercise does not suggest you should lie on the couch and meditate during the time you usually run or play tennis.

You are looking for balance. You have entered into pregnancy in a strange, high-tech way, but now your body is finally doing something it was made to do: grow a baby. If you eat a good diet, get adequate rest, exercise in moderation and take prenatal vitamins, you will be doing what you can to give your baby a good start in life. Remember that it will be good for you and for the baby to regard this pregnancy as a natural process rather than as a scientific project.

How much will this baby be "mine"?

All parents have ideas of what their children will be like. Most base these expectations on their own appearance, interests and abilities. Tall parents expect tall children, engineers expect little engineers, women with curls expect babies with curls, and neatness is expected to beget neatness. Rarely, if ever, do parents get the children about whom they fantasize. Almost always, parents come to accept and often celebrate the ways their real children differ from their fantasy children.

Women who know their donors inevitably assume that their children will resemble the donor in some way. After all, if you didn't expect the donor's appearance, intelligence, personality and health to express themselves in the child, you wouldn't care where the egg came from. But you do care and you do expect to see the donor in your child. If she is your sister, this will generate one set of feelings, and if she is someone you found through a donor agency, selected from her pictures and questionnaire and met only once, other feelings will arise.

What if you never met your donor? Never spoke with her by phone? Although openness is becoming increasingly common, there remain many women who carry babies created from the eggs of strangers. If the donor is a stranger, you may wonder if the baby, also, will feel like a stranger. One woman, who had a child from a donated egg several years ago and never saw a photo of the donor, recalls having images of something out of the movie *Alien*. The film was popular at the time and she remembers thinking that an alien would "pop out of my stomach."

Women pregnant with a child through egg donation often describe going through a process of questioning the "mine-ness" of their baby. They describe wondering, especially at the beginning of the pregnancy, whether this can really be their baby. Fortunately, this question, which can be torturous for some, seems to diminish over time.

In the words of Sandra, 38 and an expectant mom:

> Mother has taken on a whole new wonderful meaning for me. It is not about conceiving anymore. It is not about genes. It's about

nurturing a child, it's about my blood supply, what I eat, how my body takes care of the child growing within it. Yes, this will be my child.

The abundance of recent articles on epigenetics are a source of comfort and encouragement to many moms through egg donation. Epigentics confirms that if you are pregnant through egg donation, you are not simply the oven. You play an active role in shaping who your child is in ways that seem to go beyond what you eat and don't eat, drink and don't drink. Your child will be influenced by the sound of your voice, your smell, your feelings. Knowing this, together with knowing that cells from your body cross the placenta and live on in your child and that cells from your child cross the placenta and live on in you (through microchimerism), should help to solidify your sense that this is your baby.

Marriage and family therapist Carole Lieber Wilkins observes, "Mother and father and *parent* are verbs as well as nouns. We become a parent by parenting. A father is only a dad when he fathers, not when he donates sperm."

The Chinese have a belief in "the red thread." They believe that there is an invisible red thread that connects people who belong together. When people comment that your child looks like you, they are saying, as much as anything else, that you belong together. I (Ellen) have seen this in my work with adoptive parents. I have had Caucasian parents with Chinese children who tell me that people comment on how their daughter looks like them, and I can remember one fair-haired mother of a dark-skinned child from Colombia who said that other parents in her daughter's third-grade class were surprised to hear she joined their family through adoption. "But she looks just like you," this mom remembers them saying. What these comments do, we believe, is reaffirm the bonds of family and the "rightness" of particular people being together.

Bonding through the donor

Whether the donor is a sister, a friend or a stranger you have met once, your positive feelings about her will help you bond in utero with your child. Shelley Smith, Founder and Director of the Egg Donor program in Los Angeles, observes, "I see people falling in love with their donors and then, when they become pregnant, their hearts expand to love their unborn child as well" (Smith 2004).

But what about expectant moms who don't get to meet their donors? How does the anonymity of their situation impact bonding? It seems that the most important ingredient is positive feelings about the donor. You don't have to meet her to feel that she is a really good person and for you to feel your child is coming from a good place.

> I loved the way she wrote about her family and particularly her close relationship with her sister. There were other prospective donors who looked more like me, but we chose this particular donor because family is so important to me and this was something I wanted to have in common with her. (Helena, 43 and six months pregnant)

Privacy issues

When you are in the midst of infertility treatment, you give up all privacy. As Lucy, 33, put it when she was introduced to yet another physician in her infertility clinic, "Now I guess there is no one left in all of Minneapolis who has not seen my vagina!"

Her comment illustrates two things: women, in particular, feel as if they are surrendering all physical privacy when going through infertility treatment. The other message she conveys is that it helps to keep laughing!

Being pregnant means being very public about a very private matter: you are having a baby. Being pregnant with a donated egg raises new questions of privacy. Does anyone need to know the origins of your pregnancy? If so, who?

If you are newly pregnant through egg donation, your challenge comes in claiming your right to privacy but distinguishing it from secrecy. We would venture to say that there is no reason why you should feel compelled to tell people who comment on your pregnancy or congratulate you, how you conceived. It is simply a private matter. Does the woman next to you in prenatal yoga class or the couple you stop to talk with on the way out of your childbirth class need to know? Would you be inclined to tell them other private information?

> Karen, 40, pregnant with a donated egg, told her family she was pregnant. When her father asked, "Is it donor egg?" she replied, "Does it really matter?" Her father said, "No," and discussion ended there.

On the other hand, your obstetrician and your child's pediatrician should know the origins of the pregnancy. Why? Because the physician who treats you will make certain assumptions based on who you are and on your health. For example, the physician who recommends an amnio because you are 40 years old would probably have a different recommendation if you told him/her your pregnancy came from eggs of a donor who was under 30. Similarly, the pediatrician will seek family medical history in order to offer informed care for his/her new little patient. You will want to explain to the pediatrician that you are providing your donor's medical history. Don't be surprised, however, if he (or she) also wants some medical history on your side as well. As an adoptive mother, I (Ellen) once had that experience and asked the physician about it. He answered that he feels environment, nutrition and lifestyle all influence health and disease.

Ambivalence

Ambivalence is a natural part of becoming a parent, and when pregnancy comes easily, most expectant parents are not shy about acknowledging some ambivalence. However, it is much more difficult to acknowledge mixed feelings when you have worked so hard to become pregnant. I (Ellen) have a client who is 18 weeks pregnant through egg donation after many years of effort and countless pregnancy losses along the way. It has not been an easy pregnancy so far and my client has suffered from severe nausea and fatigue. However, perhaps her greatest suffering comes in the form of guilt: she reluctantly admits to me that "I'm not liking this baby very much." To this I respond, "How could you? The baby has taken over your body and wreaked havoc on your life." To this, my patient breathes a visible sigh of relief and smiles.

Infertile couples, in general, feel they have no right to feel ambivalent. Years ago, there was an ad for Toyota automobiles that said, "You wanted it, you got it, Toyota." In those days there were a fair number of people pregnant after infertility nicknaming their growing fetuses "Toyota." They wanted it, they got it…there was nothing to complain about.

Egg donation leaves even less room for ambivalence. Seeking and securing an egg donor and going through all that is involved in terms of time, energy, finances and, above all, emotional gymnastics leaves people little room to think, "I'm not sure" or "Maybe I don't want to do this after all."

Ambivalence is part of pregnancy. It is also part of parenthood. We expect that you will adore and cherish the child you give birth to, but there will be moments (maybe hours or even days) when you wonder, "Was it really worth it?" or think wistfully of the days when you had the freedom to do whatever you wanted without thinking about childcare, naps, school vacation schedules and the lot.

Learning whether it is a boy or a girl—or both

We live in a time in which many pregnant women know the gender of their child or twins prior to birth. Ultrasounds not only make it easy to learn this information but they make it somewhat difficult *not* to learn it.

With all you have been through, you may want the surprise of not knowing the gender of your child. You may feel that not knowing is one opportunity to return to the old-fashioned, natural way of having a baby. With all the high-tech interventions, it may feel comforting to look away from the ultrasound screen and ask that medical personnel not tell you whether you are having a boy or a girl.

Or you may feel otherwise. If choosing egg donation was a complicated and challenging decision, you may have strong feelings about whether it will be easier to have a boy or a girl. Some women pregnant through egg donation feel that if they have a girl, they will share more with her and feel a sense of closeness that will compensate or partially compensate for the loss of a genetic connection. Or they may feel that a boy will be easier because many boys have a "special thing" for their mothers.

If you already have a child—especially a full biological child— you may hope for a child of the opposite gender, feeling that this may make things easier in many ways. You can still opt to not know the gender, but you may feel that you want to be prepared and that knowing the gender will help you prepare your older child for the arrival of a baby sister or brother.

The important thing is not whether you learn the gender or not but that you take some control of the situation and let your preferences be known. Having endured—and benefitted from— so much medical intervention, it is important that you feel a right to speak up and control the flow of information about your child's gender. This includes making the choice to know yourselves but not to tell family members and friends.

Finding support

Some women pregnant through egg donation say, "I don't feel part of the fertile world or the infertility world—I just feel different." You may actually find that relationships established with other infertile couples whom you have met throughout your journey are threatened with the news of your pregnancy. On the other hand, maybe you and your infertile friends have found ways to talk openly and honestly along the way about the complex feelings that arise when one person becomes pregnant and another does not.

You are likely to encounter some mixed experiences with your infertile friends. Some, who are just beginning to contemplate egg donation, may be inspired by your pregnancy and credit you with helping them consider this option. Others, who don't like the idea of egg donation or, more likely, are not ready to think about it, may pull back. This can be hurtful, but remember that friendships that are worth having will survive the stresses and strains of infertility and pregnancy.

Finding a pediatrician

Yes, if this is your first child, you will need to find a pediatrician. This should not be a difficult task logistically, since pediatrics seems to attract some of the kindest and most approachable physicians. Good pediatricians, with privileges at good hospitals, abound. Nonetheless, it may not feel so easy to make a few calls so that you can visit a few pediatric offices.

You may feel that you are being presumptuous calling a pediatrician before you have a baby. If you have had pregnancy losses along the way, it may be especially difficult. Remind yourself that this is how it's done—expectant parents (and you are one of them!) do contact pediatricians several months before their due dates. After all, the pediatrician will need to examine your baby shortly after birth.

What to look for

- Your pediatrician should be affiliated with a hospital or medical center with an excellent pediatrics department.

- Your pediatrician should have a well-staffed office that you can get into and out of without expecting to wait hours in the waiting room.

- Your pediatrician or his/her staff should be available for a call back for an urgent phone call.

- Your pediatrician should have a nursing staff that is accessible, answers questions and helps you with routine concerns.

Most importantly, you should be able to talk comfortably from the start about donor conception. You should tell prospective doctors your history on first meeting. Doing so will accomplish two things: first, you will know, right then and there, if this is someone you can feel comfortable with; second, you won't have a secret that you might someday have to reveal to your doctor.

Childbirth

We wish that every expectant mom could plan her labor and delivery and have it go the way she wants. We would wish this all the more for moms through egg donation. You went through a lot to have this baby and now you face more unknowns. Will your labor be short or long, easy or hard? Will you be able to deliver vaginally or will you need a Caesarean section?

Infertility prepared you well for childbirth. You learned, long ago, that you can't plan for your delivery. That said, there are a few things you can do to help ensure that things go as closely as they can to the way you would want them to.

Educate yourself—in childbirth classes and through talking with your physician and nurses—about the options for childbirth. When can a midwife deliver your baby? Does your physician and his/her hospital have a high rate of C-sections? How and why is it decided that a section is necessary? What options are there for reducing pain?

Make sure your husband/partner knows what you want—it can be difficult making decisions when you are in labor and in pain.

Breastfeeding

Breastfeeding is a personal decision. There is ample medical evidence that it promotes good health in your infant and evidence as well that it is beneficial for moms, too. And many women pregnant through egg donation feel strongly that they want to breastfeed because it is another important physical connection they will have with their child. All that said, breastfeeding may not be for you.

Once again our focus is on you feeling in charge of your decision making. There is no absolute right or wrong with this decision: the important thing is that you make the decision that is best for you and your new family.

Some tips for when you are pregnant

Preserving memories

Making regular entries into a journal can be helpful in several ways. For one, it will give you a place to put thoughts and feelings. This will help you preserve memories you don't want to lose and to organize feelings that may seem scattered and intense. You can record them, read them over a day or week or month later and, perhaps, see them from a different perspective. Your journal can also serve as a repository of information that you might otherwise risk losing. For example, if you have a meeting with your donor, you can record specific information she gives you about her history and that of her family, and you can preserve a description of your meeting—where you met, what you thought when you saw her, how you felt sitting there and talking with someone who was giving you such an incredible gift.

Remember that children love to hear stories about themselves and, in particular, the story of how they were born. Photos make it even more fun. For parents concerned about how their child will make sense of it all, what could be better than having a visual diary of your journey to parenthood through egg donation? Take photos of the people at the program, meetings with the donor if you do this, a visit to the donor's city. Keep copies of ultrasounds.

Before and during your pregnancy, obtain as much information as you can about your donor. Make sure that photos, a biography, letters and all else that you can gather are duplicated and kept in two places—a safe deposit box or something else that is completely secure—and someplace easily accessible in your home.

Psychologist Maggie Kirkman, PhD, a researcher at the Key Centre for Women's Health in Society at the University of Melbourne in Australia, advises parents to make a book about each of their donor-conceived children as a contribution to explaining their origins and to developing their own stories. She recommends accompanying photographs, with a text that emphasizes how much the parents wanted a baby and how happy the birth as made them. It can explain that all babies need an egg and sperm to grow and that Mum had no eggs. The story of finding the donor can be told, as well as the role of the doctor in putting the egg and sperm together. Kansas social worker Kris Probasco describes a similar project and calls it a Beginnings Book. Probasco observes that children use these books over the years to gain understanding of their origins and to put the pieces together. Kirkman observes that the book encourages children to take the initiative in talking about their own stories and to indulge in the repetition that children enjoy; it is a fixed point to which they can refer when matters become confused; it can give children pleasure and reassurance to see their own name and story in a book; and it has a status of legitimacy, like other books, that oral accounts may lack. This may not work for all parents or all children, but it is a technique that several families in her research found to be helpful.

Take lots of pictures of yourself (or your partner) pregnant

For moms through egg donation, the profoundly intimate experience of pregnancy is of paramount importance, and photos of that experience can be validating and affirming. You and your child will be physically connected from the time the embryo(s) is transferred to you. The pictures taken of you with your child growing inside you will provide wonderful memories of your union.

Find some traveling companions

It will be helpful for you to know other women who are pregnant, especially others who are pregnant through egg donation. You may have made some friends in a support group or from your physician's waiting room and be pregnant at the same time as some of them. If this isn't the case, we encourage you to reach out. There are online support groups (complete with virtual showers!) and groups through RESOLVE, the American Fertility Association, the Donor Conception Network (UK), Access A (Australia), the Infertility Awareness Association (Canada) and others worldwide.

Do not feel that you need to limit yourself to groups made up only of others pregnant with donor eggs or pregnant after infertility. Although it may be frustrating to hear other women worrying about stretch marks or complaining about how much weight they've gained, this is normal pregnancy talk, and yours is a normal pregnancy. You may not always feel it, but you have finally joined the club.

Multiple gestation

"Not me," you think. "Not us. We're so infertile, we could never have twins." Indeed, most women who become pregnant with donated eggs carry singleton pregnancies, but even as physicians work actively to limit the number of embryos transferred, there remain many twin pregnancies and some triplets as well. According to the US Center for Disease Control 2008 statistics, of the 6843 pregnancies in the US using fresh embryos with donor eggs, 39 percent were twins and 3 percent were triplets or more.

When you were approaching egg donation, you probably had feelings about whether you wanted to have twins. For some intended parents, exhausted and daunted by the costs of egg donation, the prospect of instant family or "two for the price of one" is appealing. However, for others, a twin pregnancy, which brings risks of prematurity, is frightening. Some intended parents are so concerned that they made sure their doctor transferred only one embryo. Others feel that, given all they'd been through and the costs involved, they were willing to accept the risk of a twin pregnancy.

We hope that if you wanted one, you got one, and that if you wanted two, you are carrying twins. However, this is not always the case. We have known women who found themselves envying fellow travelers who are having twins and feeling guilty for "not being grateful for what we have." We've also known a number of newly pregnant moms who have gone into panic mode when they learn that it is a twin pregnancy. If you are newly pregnant, take some time to let the news settle in.

Even if you thought this through carefully, surprises can still happen. This can occur if one embryo splits, creating identical twins, or if there is, for some reason, a change of plans at the last minute and a third embryo is transferred. Therapist Carole Lieber Wilkins reports that some of the women she has worked with who have had triplet or higher pregnancies found themselves in very difficult positions on the morning of the embryo transfer. At a time of heightened anxiety and on medications that affected their mood, many had to make a decision about "that extra embryo that doesn't look good."

"The physician will suggest 'we put it in anyway' because it looks 'bad,' and then that embryo ends up being the triplet or the quad," Lieber Wilkins says. She encourages her patients to be conservative and to consider hypothetical situations in advance.

Multiple pregnancy—maintaining privacy

To the extent that women pregnant with donated eggs wish to maintain some privacy, a multiple gestation challenges this. Twin pregnancies generate questions about the use of fertility drugs, and once the babies are born, all the more attention comes your way. Strangers on the street or in the supermarket have no qualms about asking you if you took fertility medications. And even those who refrain from such intrusive comments feel fully entitled to comment on the twins, to ask how old they are or where they were born or how you manage with two. Such questions have nothing to do with egg donation, but they are an intrusion on your privacy.

> Natalie, 42, was self-conscious about the fact that her twins did not look like her in any way. People often commented on this, and when they did, she often felt that they were "suspecting it was egg donation." Although it was difficult, the mom was able to handle these incidents. Then something happened which proved much more challenging. "I went to a store and a woman said, 'Are they yours?' I was used to that and had learned to simply smile and say a proud, 'Yes.' But the woman went on and said, 'Your grandchildren are beautiful.' I felt like I wanted to fall off the face of the earth."

Another privacy concern comes for parents who have children through two different donors or who have a biological child and then a child through egg donation. Parents worry that if their children look different from one another and people take note of it (which they inevitably do), the family's privacy will be repeatedly challenged. Remember that even within "regular" biological families, siblings often look very different from one another. When people comment on these differences, they are simply making superficial observations, and there is no need to respond to them with anything of substance. It is really no different, we feel, than if they were to say, "Your baby looks young to already be walking" or "Your daughter has beautiful eyes" or "Your twins look so cute sleeping next to each other." You say, "Yes" or "Okay" or "Thank you," and move on.

Pregnancy loss

"It's nature's way. It wasn't meant to be." All too often women and men who lose a pregnancy hear this pronouncement. The words sting, especially when the pregnancy, so quickly dismissed, was long-sought and deeply cherished.

Pregnancy loss after egg donation brings added dimensions of pain. In addition to the loss that any expectant parent feels when the baby who was beginning to make their heart sing is gone, parents through egg donation face an array of questions ranging from "Did we force something to happen that really was not meant to be?" and "Was I diligent enough in taking care of myself?" to "Should we try again with a different donor?" and "Can we afford to try again?" to "How much more frustration and loss can we endure?" to "Maybe it really wasn't an egg problem after all?" and "Maybe there is something so wrong with me and my body that I can't carry a baby, even with 'good' eggs?" We will briefly define the various forms of pregnancy loss.

First trimester loss

Most miscarriages occur before eight weeks of pregnancy, but since many women miscarry before they even know they are pregnant, the prevalence of early miscarriage is underreported. Current understanding is that most of the very early losses are the result of chromosomal abnormalities. Problems in the uterine environment are less often a cause of first trimester losses.

For women who become pregnant through egg donation, early loss can be very confusing, raising the question "Should we try with a different donor or was this loss a random event?"

Another form of early loss and one that is especially confusing is what is termed "biochemical pregnancy." Contrary to the old dictum "You can't be a little bit pregnant," you now learn the exact opposite: that you are "a little bit pregnant." Your first pregnancy test indicates a very low positive number and subsequent tests confirm that the pregnancy is not progressing. Physicians believe that a biochemical pregnancy occurs when an embryo stops growing and developing before it ever really implants in the uterine wall.

Second trimester loss

Late miscarriages are caused by either maternal or fetal factors. The most common cause of late miscarriage is a maternal factor involving premature dilation of the cervix, but fibroid tumors and uterine abnormalities are other maternal causes of late miscarriage.

Although most chromosomally abnormal fetuses do not survive beyond 12 weeks, some do. A fetus may appear to be developing normally but still have something inherently wrong with it which will cause it to abort. Immunological problems, related to either parent, are another possible cause of second trimester losses.

Stillbirth

A pregnancy loss after 20 weeks gestation is often referred to as a stillbirth. However, we feel that loss at 20 weeks, before viability, is very different from a loss several weeks later, at a time when a baby could live outside the womb. We will focus our discussion on loss after viability.

There are many potential causes of stillbirth. One possible loss is a malfunction in the umbilical cord, resulting in a loss of oxygen to the fetus. If the umbilical cord is compressed during the delivery, or if it becomes wrapped around the baby's neck, it can cut off the oxygen supply and result in the death of the infant.

Placental problems can also lead to intrauterine death. If the placenta is implanted too low in the uterus (placenta previa), it can separate prematurely and cause the mother to hemorrhage. Alternatively, if the baby is post-mature, the placenta may begin to malfunction, thereby depriving the baby of oxygen.

Other possible causes of stillbirth include conditions in the mother such as toxemia, diabetes or high blood pressure. Each can compromise the flow of nutrients to the baby. Or, if the mother's water breaks prematurely, the baby may contract a life-threatening infection.

Loss in multiple pregnancy

Without a doubt, a multiple pregnancy brings with it certain risks. You may experience a partial loss, either early in the pregnancy or later on. Early loss in a multiple pregnancy occurs when initial ultrasounds reveal two or more gestational sacs, but later ultrasounds fail to detect heartbeats in all of them. Often, the sac that has no heartbeat vanishes on its own. This may feel like a disenfranchised grief—you wanted one baby, you're getting one, so what are you sad about? The answer is that you are sad because your perspective changed once you learned you were carrying more than one. It is entirely natural for expectant parents to attach to the idea of twins and to want to celebrate the specialness of this pregnancy, and the excitement of an instant family.

By the second and third trimesters, expectant parents have formed bonds to each of their babies. When an ultrasound reveals that a fetus has died in utero or that it will not survive past birth because of congenital problems, this constitutes a real loss for the parents who had come to expect two babies, had begun to know two babies and were looking forward to being parents of twins.

Multifetal reduction refers to the termination of one or more fetuses in a multiple gestation. Most people who have more than two embryos transferred, whether with egg donation or not, are aware that multifetal reduction is available. However, few anticipate how painful it is for parents who worked so hard to achieve a pregnancy to elect to reduce a pregnancy from three or four to two. Only in unusual circumstances would multifetal reduction be recommended in a twin pregnancy. Although most women attempting pregnancy through egg donation have no more than two embryos transferred, there are instances in which one splits, resulting in a pregnancy composed of identical twins and a triplet. Sadly, these expectant parents, who so deeply want all their children, are forced to make the best decision they can for the future health of their babies and, often, that decision seems to be to partially reduce the pregnancy.

Sadly, there are couples who lose an entire pregnancy, often because of severe prematurity. As hard as moms-to-be work to try to delay labor, and as much as their physicians attempt to assist them in this, there are too many times when the babies simply come too early. Jean Kollantai, founder of the Center for Loss in Multiple Birth (CLIMB), a support network for parents throughout the United States and Canada who have experienced the loss of one or more fetuses during pregnancy, observes that parents who lose both their babies often feel angry at the technology that was successful in helping them conceive their children, but was unsuccessful in saving them. This loss is all the more painful when it follows a multifetal reduction, which attempted to create space for the healthy development of one or two fetuses, but which unintentionally resulted in the loss of all. Kollantai adds that some feel guilty for having wanted children so much that they turned to technology that put them at greater risk for multiple gestation.

Although we have provided some of the medical explanations for pregnancy loss, the reality is that, in many instances, it is a mystery. All too often, grieving parents are left to wonder what they could have done differently. Sadly, many blame themselves, and, perhaps to a lesser extent, their physicians. Some people blame God, wondering why they are being punished for wanting to be parents.

Questions that may arise following loss after egg donation
DID WE FORCE SOMETHING TO HAPPEN
THAT WAS NOT MEANT TO BE?

Pregnancy through egg donation is surely not a spontaneous, natural occurrence. Rather, it is the result of hard work and of advanced medical technology. While they are seeking an egg donor or attempting pregnancy after they have found her, many would-be parents wonder if what they are doing is morally right.

Sadly, women who lose a donor-egg-assisted pregnancy may be plagued by the question of whether they tried to make something happen that was "not meant to be."

WAS I DILIGENT ENOUGH IN TAKING CARE OF MYSELF?

Since it seems that any woman who loses a pregnancy looks back and scrutinizes her every action and reaction during pregnancy, it comes as no surprise that donor-egg moms-to-be are experts at self-doubt and recrimination. After all, you are the expectant moms who took self-care most seriously, having promised yourselves that you would do all you could to grow your babies well.

Unfortunately, nature has its way of making its own decisions, regardless of what you did and thought and ate. Even our brief summary of the causes of pregnancy loss reveals that many pregnancy losses, especially miscarriages early and late, are caused by problems in the fetus that have nothing to do with the maternal environment. Other losses are simply unexplained. And even those losses that can be attributed to a problem with the placenta or cervix or uterus are unrelated to your actions and reactions.

SHOULD WE TRY AGAIN WITH A DIFFERENT DONOR?

Following a few failed cycles or a pregnancy loss, people find themselves wondering if they should consider another donor. Depending upon who your donor is, how you came to enter into a donor pregnancy effort together and what your other options are, you may be more or less reluctant to think about changing donors.

If your donor is your sister or your best friend and both of you feel great about this decision, you probably won't be thinking about changing donors. In fact, you and your donor may be grieving together and trying to see this as a step forward towards your shared goal. Similarly, if your donor is someone you found through a program, met, spent time with and liked, you are probably reluctant to move on. On the other hand, if she is someone you have never met, you may feel that this pregnancy— and, perhaps, this match—wasn't meant to be.

Decisions about choosing another donor will be shaped by the nature of your pregnancy loss as well. If you have suffered an ectopic pregnancy or a loss caused by an incompetent cervix, you may feel certain that this loss had nothing to do with the donor. On the other hand, an early loss, which could be caused by chromosomal abnormalities, may prompt you to wonder about another donor.

Whatever your thoughts and whatever you decide, this will not be an easy process. No one chooses a donor—whether family member or friend—without careful thought, exploration and discussion. By the time you start a cycle with a given donor, you will have already begun to bond with the idea of a baby conceived with this donor's egg. Having actually experienced a pregnancy through her eggs has only served to solidify your dream of a baby created with her egg, your partner's sperm and your love.

Can we afford to try again?

As we see throughout this book, cost plays a huge role in some decision making about using donor eggs and a negligible one in others. Differences are tied not only to family finances and to whether you have a volunteer donor or not, but also to insurance coverage for egg donation.

If you are self-paying for your medical treatment and for the donor, the costs of doing another cycle are high. You might have decided, prior to treatment, that you could only afford one cycle—that some financial resources had to be left in place for adoption if the cycle didn't work. However, now you have had a pregnancy and, if it was an early loss, you may feel, "We got one step closer to our goal; we can't quit now." You may find yourselves in a real dilemma: not wanting to commit money you may later need for adoption, but reluctant to give up on egg donation when you now know that you can achieve pregnancy.

How much frustration and loss can we endure?

Here it is, the question that runs through all infertility treatment: "When is enough enough?" Couples who have never conceived ask this question, and couples who have recurrent miscarriages ask it, as do those who don't conceive with donated gametes and those who have pregnancy loss after gamete donation. How do people know when they have reached their limit, when they are simply putting good money and good time and energy after bad?

In talking with countless couples facing the question "When is enough enough?" I (Ellen) have developed a profound respect for people's ability to know when the time has come to move on. It may sound simplistic, but people have a way of knowing. Sometimes that knowing comes because one or both members of a couple realizes that he/she simply has to stop—the person has run out of steam, of hope and belief. Other times, someone feels they have been given a sign. For example, I (Ellen) had a client, a physician, who found herself treating a very sick woman who worked in adoption, specifically with China. My client, deep in the throes of IVF, remembers thinking, "Now it has come together—I am going to save her life and she is going to help me get a baby."

Maybe it wasn't an egg problem after all?

What a thorny question this is. Again, it is one of the questions that concern only some couples who suffer pregnancy loss after egg donation. Spared this question are those of you who know—for sure—that you need donated eggs in order to conceive, as well as those whose pregnancy loss appeared entirely unrelated to egg quality.

But what about those who turned to egg donation because of unexplained infertility and have now had an early loss? More frustration. Sadly, you have no way of knowing whether your loss was simply a random event—which it probably was—or whether the real problem may be uterine or male factor. At this juncture, you will probably want to talk with your physician to see what he recommends about exploring uterine factors or, possibly, introducing donor sperm with your eggs, assuming you, as a couple, are comfortable with parenthood through sperm donation. Depending on your stamina and on the accessibility of other medical treatment, you may also want to seek a second opinion. We are not suggesting that you keep yourselves on an endless pursuit of pregnancy, but we do want you to avoid the painful regret that so often comes when people look back and question, "Did we do all that we could?"

MAYBE THERE IS SOMETHING SO WRONG WITH ME AND MY BODY THAT I CAN'T CARRY A BABY EVEN WITH GOOD EGGS?
How very, very sad that people sometimes get the message that "all you need are good eggs." And so we remind you, yet again, that reproduction is a mystery. This really isn't about there being something wrong with you, and, most likely, it's not something wrong with your body. Even today, with all the recent advances in reproductive medicine, so much remains unanswered about conception and pregnancy.

Grief, mourning and moving on

Whatever form the loss takes—and we again acknowledge that there are enormous differences between early miscarriage and full-term stillbirth—grieving parents need to mourn the loss of the child they were expecting before taking steps to bring another child into the family. This will be all the more true for those of you who decide to move on to adoption, since you will be grieving not only the child you have lost but also the opportunity to share pregnancy, childbirth and partial genetic connection. However, it is also true for those of you who suffered an early loss. Even if you are optimistically resuming efforts with the same donor, there has been a loss. You were expecting a particular baby, you were beginning to imagine him, to name him, to become excited about being pregnant.

Once again, we turn our attention to the particulars of egg donation. How does the fact that your pregnancy was donor-assisted impact your loss and help shape your grieving process?

Shared grief

If your donor is your sister or your close friend, she is likely to be part of your grief process. Although the magnitude of your loss is different, she, too, has lost something. She went through a great deal to help you achieve pregnancy and she was invested in its outcome. We hope that the camaraderie you feel with her softens your grief rather than intensifies it.

Complicated mourning

Psychologists and others who offer counsel around grief and mourning have long noted that grief becomes more complicated and challenging when the mourner has had an ambivalent relationship with the person or role that has been lost. Such may be the case with pregnancy loss after egg donation—the pregnancy was most often deeply wanted, but it was also the source of some ambivalence. In addition to the normal ambivalence that many pregnant women feel when a little person invades their body, women pregnant with donated eggs arrive with a complicated history. There may have been earlier pregnancy losses, perhaps with one's own eggs, or uncertainty about trying donor eggs.

Rituals

Few established rituals and ceremonies exist for early pregnancy loss. Sadly, even late losses are sometimes dismissed as unworthy of a funeral and burial. Hence, many grieving parents, whether their pregnancy was conceived spontaneously, through their own gametes and ART or with donor gametes, feel that theirs is a disenfranchised grief. All too often, the rest of the world pours salt in their wounds by saying, "At least you know you can get pregnant" or "It wasn't meant to be" or, worse still, "Do you think you should quit your job next time and just rest?"

The absence of rituals and public acknowledgement of loss is complicated for egg donation parents since many felt very private when they were pregnant. Hesitant to tell people about the pregnancy until it was well established, some of you may have suffered your loss before others even knew you were expecting. Others may have told people you were pregnant, but still handled the pregnancy with circumspection and ever a keen eye on privacy. Now you long for others to acknowledge your loss and to honor the memory of the child or children you were expecting. The distance you understandably maintained during the weeks or months you were pregnant may make it all the more difficult for others to reach out to you now, especially in the absence of a memorial service or other observance of your loss.

We encourage you to create your own rituals. You may want to talk with a clergyperson for some assistance or with a professional at a funeral home. Or you may feel comfortable creating your own ritual. Some grieving parents have planted trees, written goodbye letters to their lost child(ren) or donated children's books to a local library or goods to an orphanage. Some have stood at water's edge and recited a prayer or a poem. Others have created a gravestone to capture their feelings towards the child they lost. One especially moving stone had an etching of a small angel with the words "If love had been enough to save you, you would have lived."

The odds are with you

Although loss is possible, it is not probable. If you conceive through egg donation, the greatest likelihood is that you will deliver a healthy baby. You may have been told that you had a 60–70 percent chance of becoming pregnant; once pregnancy is achieved, the odds shift dramatically in your favor. And they improve as time goes on—when you are six weeks pregnant you may be told that you have a 85 percent or so chance of taking a baby home, but by 12 weeks the percentage is probably in the high 90s. So when you are pregnant with your donor-egg-conceived child, we encourage you to look forward, not back, and to begin to anticipate the arrival of your much wanted and long sought-after child. You are pregnant. Life is growing inside you. This, as you know all too well, is a glorious achievement. Take some time to celebrate.

– 8 –

Parenthood after Egg Donation

Parenthood is filled with countless tasks, rewards, delights and challenges, most of which have nothing to do with how your child joined your family. Being the kindergarten room parent or the tooth fairy, helping with homework, doing piles of camp laundry or planning a birthday party are all unrelated to conception. You don't need this book to know about these joys and tasks of parenthood. Here we focus on thoughts and feelings related to egg donation.

Your parenting partnership

When first thinking about egg donation, many couples worry that they will experience an inequality since the father will have a genetic connection to their child and the mother will not. We have found that fears of inequality rarely materialize. For one thing, the experience of going through infertility treatment and making decisions about egg donation often fortifies a couple and helps prepare them to be an effective parenting team. In addition, pregnancy validates a woman's central role in bringing her child into the world. After caring for her child in utero and delivering her baby, it is hard for a new mom to see her husband as the more authentic parent.

Many moms through egg donation say that they feel proud and happy to have had their husband's child. Fathers express admiration for their wives, who so often endured years of intrusive infertility treatments before pregnancy through egg donation.

Still, there are ways in which new parents are challenged. In addition to all the normal stresses of having an infant—sleep deprivation, piles of laundry, added expenses and loss of time to oneself—there are some additional challenges that may arise after egg donation.

First, you may be the parents of twins. While the arrival of twins often feels like a special reward for years of infertility, it is an exhausting time. One or both of your twins may have spent days, weeks—or longer—in the neonatal intensive care unit (NICU). You may have gone home with both babies remaining in the hospital or you may take one home before the other, leaving you juggling your time between home and the NICU. Even when both babies are at home, it is exhausting: just when you have fed or diapered or bathed one, the other needs your attention. The seemingly endless needs of two newborns are stressful on any couple. Having wanted your children so much and worked so hard to have them, there is additional stress: it feels hard to complain or express frustration to yourself, let alone to your partner.

Next, you have gone from being child-LESS to being parents. We emphasize the LESS part of things because your experience has been different from your fertile friends. In many instances, they married, took some time to enjoy being child-free and then had their first child. For you, there may have been years of infertility or, if you married when you were older, pressured attempts to become parents soon after you became a couple. Either way, you are not coming off a lovely stretch of child-free living. You are emerging from a very stressful time that was followed by the stresses of the egg donation process, pregnancy and, possibly, multiple gestation.

Then there is the matter of division of labor. Like all new parents, you will have to figure out who does what when it comes to feeding and diapering your baby, laundry, shopping and all the tasks that increase exponentially with the arrival of an infant. This can feel more complicated for parents after egg donation because of what you went through to become parents. You probably tried your best to share the burdens of infertility treatment and pregnancy, but it is the new mother who is the veteran of years of injections, blood tests, early morning ultrasounds. You may have endured multiple miscarriages. And now you have successfully accomplished nine months of pregnancy, complete with fatigue, nausea, uncomfortable weight gain, possibly back aches and so on. It may feel just a bit unfair when your husband wants a Saturday afternoon off to play golf or when he expects you to figure out childcare. There may be spoken—or unspoken—feelings that he has had it easy: he went through a lot less physically and he got to have a child he is genetically connected to.

We have no magic formula for how to address the dynamics of your parenting partnership, but we encourage you to be aware that new parenthood is incredibly stressful and all the more so when it comes after a long struggle with infertility or pregnancy losses. Be sure, from the start, to tend to your relationship. This means finding the time to be together as a couple, both at home and going out. Part of your job as new parents is to identify some trusted babysitters and, once you have them on board, plan date nights and, before too much time passes, even an overnight away. Remember that the best gift you can give your child or children is the opportunity to grow up with parents who love and respect each other.

Talking with others about donor conception

If you are a new parent through egg donation, we hope you feel proud and happy about how you built your family. You made decisions carefully and worked hard to achieve your goal. You have nothing to be ashamed of—no secrets to keep. Still, there is the matter of privacy. You can't help but wonder, "Who should know our child was born through egg donation?" "What should we say to them and when should we say it?"

We approach this topic from the dual perspectives of "need to know" and "reason to know." There are a few people who absolutely need to know about donor conception. We include in this category your child, any other children in the family, your obstetrician, your child's pediatrician and any other medical professionals involved in your child's care. We add close family members who may not need to know about donor conception when you are pregnant or right after the child is born, but will need to know at some point because you will want your child feeling comfortable talking openly about his origins.

So who is in the "reason to know" category? These are the folks in your lives that you do not have an absolute obligation to tell but whom you may choose to tell because you conclude there is a reason to tell them. Here are some examples of people in the "reason to tell" category.

Close friends

There are many reasons why you might want to tell your close friends you chose egg donation. For one thing, we hope you will feel pleased and proud of the choices you made, and most of us like to share these kinds of feelings with friends. In addition, your friends may well have been part of your infertility journey. If this is the case—if you talked with them about your struggles and your treatment—you may now feel that you are being secretive if you neglect to mention that you chose egg donation.

People you know who are considering egg donation

There may be people you meet or know who are considering egg donation. Although you would not otherwise volunteer to them how your pregnancy occurred, this information becomes relevant if they bring up the topic of egg donation. For example, I (Ellen) have a client who was having dinner with a friend who is the mother of two children, five and seven. My client told her friend she was considering egg donation, to which the friend replied, "That's great—my kids were born through egg donation." Initially, my client was stunned, wondering why her friend had never told her this before. Then she understood: there had never before been a reason to tell and now there was.

Circumstances in which the subject of egg donation arises

The topic of egg donation rarely arises in daily life. When you go to the dry cleaner or sign your child up for violin lessons or take a yoga class, no one is likely to be talking about egg donation. But what about a mother-of-twins group? I (Ellen) know a mom through egg donation who went to a mother-of-twins group because she wanted to hear how other women were managing to care for two babies at the same time. She had no intention of saying that her twins came from egg donation, but when the other women went around the group to introduce themselves, a few of them made note of the fact that they had used egg donation. Once the topic was raised, my client felt that it was appropriate for her to also acknowledge that egg donation was part of her history.

People you simply feel like telling

Another reason to tell is that you *want* to. You are talking with a friend or an acquaintance or a total stranger and something prompts you to tell your story. You are not telling someone in a self-conscious way but coming rather from a place of pride and confidence. Something has reminded you of your good fortune, of what a miracle your family is, and you want to share your great pleasure with another person. You have the strong feeling that your story will touch this person's heart. Carrie, the mother of twins through egg donation, says that as time goes on she finds herself telling more and more people.

> It's something I'm proud about and I want people to know this. I always get positive reactions and sometimes there is a special connect. I've had someone thank me and tell me that her daughter is struggling with infertility. I've had childless women say they wish this option had been available to them.

Medical specialists

We advised earlier that your child's pediatrician will *need* to know about donor conception. Although much of pediatric care has nothing to do with family history, certain conditions, illnesses and traits have hereditary components. You will want your child's physician to be basing his/her care of your child on an accurate family history. But what about other medical specialists? We suppose that if your child breaks his arm, the orthopedic surgeon doesn't really need to know about egg donation. However, when anesthesia and medications are involved, it seems safest to provide all physicians with as much information as possible.

Does your child's dentist need to know that your child was created through egg donation? It may become a good idea. Although brushing and flossing habits are not hereditary, family history can be relevant in other aspects of dental medicine. These can include use of medications and anesthesia, which are needed for dental surgery.

Teachers

Is there any reason that a teacher would need to know that your child was conceived through egg donation? We can think of one: elementary school units on the family. In the early school years there are often class discussions of family formation. Adoptive parents have worked hard to sensitize teachers and other educators to the fact that there are many ways to form a family, a message that has been further communicated by single parents and gay and lesbian parents. Adoptive parents have also succeeded, in many school systems, in eliminating the often troublesome Family Tree assignment and having it replaced with something more akin to a "family orchard." Nonetheless, your child may be in a first- or second-grade class in which the teacher asks, "Did anyone join their family through adoption?" or "Does anyone here have a step-father or a half-sister?" Since it is possible that your confident little son or daughter may proudly raise a hand to say, "My Aunt Pat gave my mommy and daddy an egg," you might want to talk with a primary grade teacher about egg donation.

Clergy

Does your priest, minister or rabbi have reason to know that your child was conceived with donated eggs? Your response to this question has a lot to do with your relationship with your clergyperson. If you don't have a religious connection or are only an occasional participant in your congregation, you won't be thinking about talking with clergy about egg donation. However, if this is someone you are close with, and especially if you are planning some religious celebration such as a baby naming or a baptism, you may (or may not) want your clergy to know the special way you became a family.

If your child grows up in a religious community, he may someday want to talk with clergy about his origins. Donor conception may feel very relevant, for example, to an 11- or 12-year-old preparing to become a bar or bat mitzvah, since this service often makes reference to ancestry. However, this event comes at a time when it should be your child's decision—not yours—whether to talk.

Talking with children about reproduction and about how they entered your family

"What will we say to our child?" "When is a good time to talk with our child?" "How will we handle his questions?" "Will this information upset her, cause her to distance herself from me?"

These are but a few of the questions that parents through egg donation ask themselves. Do not let these questions morph into worries. Remember what we learned from the researchers at Emory University about the ways in which family narratives build self-esteem (Bohanek, Marin, Fivush and Duke 2006). Hearing about their parents' struggles, as well as triumphs, helps young people feel grounded in their families and clearer about their own unfolding identities.

You have a story to tell that you should feel proud of. Yours is a story of being able to ask for help and of being blessed that help was offered. Yours is a story about being flexible and resilient and able to transform a second choice into a best option. Yours is a story filled with important lessons for a child and it is ultimately a happy story. Remember also, that children love to hear about themselves. They are curious about pregnancy and they thrive in knowing how much you wanted them and how happy they made you when they finally arrived.

Your child doesn't have to fully understand what you are saying, but he does need to know that you are speaking openly, honestly and with words that reflect your great love for him and your delight in being his parent.

So where do you begin? After talking with countless parents through egg donation, as well as child psychologists, developmental specialists and adoption professionals, we encourage you to do the following.

Build your family story with confidence from the beginning

Unlike adoptive parents, whose child has an earlier story for which the parents have no authorship, with egg donation you are present at the creation. From the time you first set out to find a donor, you are creating and building your family story. We encourage you to do so with an eye on what this story will mean for your child. You will want to build a story that you can tell with pride and confidence. This may mean making decisions that are initially difficult for you. For example, some people who are hesitant or fearful about meeting their donor will push themselves to do so because they will have a more complete story for their child. Some who might have preferred a donor who had donated before will go with a first-time donor because they feel that their child is more likely to understand her donation as a gift.

Chicago therapist Judy Calica reminds us that all parents, including donor parents, want their children to have a full and authentic sense of themselves. Open, honest conversations with their parents that include full and accurate information can only help reinforce a child's sense of authenticity and wholeness.

Kansas City social worker Kris Probasco encourages her clients to create a "Beginnings Book." In it are photos of the donor and her family, the parents, the doctor/medical staff, the clinic and Kris, who often serves as their guide and advisor. Her clients follow these photos with month-by-month pregnancy photos and labor and delivery. Probasco says that having a Beginnings Book enables the children to put the pieces together. Since most of her clients have known donations that include ongoing relationships with the donor and her family, the child knows these special friends from an early age. Seeing the donor and her family in the Beginnings Book helps the child make the connection that their special friends and their family helper are one and the same.

Begin to talk about donor conception when your child is very young—before he can understand

Why do we advise this? What sense does it make to tell a child something he can't understand? We believe in early telling for a few reasons. First, it offers the child the opportunity to grow up always knowing. Instead of having to sit the child down at an older age and try to explain something that is likely to surprise or confuse your child, you have the chance to introduce the information in a natural way. Remember that the central message of this story is one that applies to most children: "Mommy and Daddy (or Mommy and Mommy or Daddy and Daddy) wanted to have a baby and were so happy to be able to have you."

Children love to hear about themselves and most are curious about pregnancy. Why not use this as an opportunity to introduce the donor. Say something like "Do you want to see pictures of when you were in my belly? I was sooooooo excited to be pregnant and I couldn't wait to meet you. Daddy and I were so happy that Samantha helped us." Your young child will have no idea who Samantha is or how she helped you, but what he will hear and understand is that you were thrilled that this precious, cherished child was on the way. Contrast this to sitting a nine- or ten- or 11-year-old down and saying, "We have something to tell you…"

Los Angeles marriage and family therapist Carole Lieber Wilkins advises the parents she works with to tell their children by the time they are three years old:

> The reason for telling a child about a third party reproduction is not because they need to know the technical details of how in vitro fertilization or inseminations were performed; it is because children need to begin the process of acknowledging that there is another person or people in the world to whom they are connected in a significant and lasting way. (lafamilybuilding.com)

Lieber Wilkins goes on to say that it is normal for children to "fantasize about the pieces of the puzzle that may not be filled in for many years" (ibid) but adds that this is not a reason to delay talking with them when they are very young. To those parents who say they are anxious about talking with their child, Lieber Wilkins recommends practice. Talking to themselves and to one another, before their child can possibly understand, helps parents find language with which they can feel comfortable and enables parents to deal with the feelings that arise at a time and in a context that feels safe.

Although most parents through egg donation subscribe to the recommendation that they begin conversations about donor conception when their children are young, there are some who wait to talk with their children. These include parents who were advised to wait, parents who kept postponing the conversation, and I (Ellen) know one family in which the parents "kept forgetting" to tell. Whatever the reason that conversations didn't begin earlier, it is important that you not get into a self-blame game. If you find yourself beginning your conversations with your teenager, so be it. Remember that you did the best you could at the time and you are where you are now for reasons. Dr. Joann Paley Galst, psychologist and co-author of *Ethical Dilemmas in Fertility Counseling*, tells the poignant story of a mom through egg donation who came to a support group where most of the other attendees were pregnant or the parents of young children. She spoke poignantly of her struggle of waiting too long and said that it became more and more difficult for her to begin the conversation as her daughter matured. She was now dealing with a mid-teens daughter who was challenging her mother with difficult questions about why she waited so long. Dr. Galst remembers the most painful part of her story being her daughter's question as to what the delay meant about how her mother felt regarding her decision to use a donor. Dr. Galst notes that there are some who advise waiting until an donor offspring is a teenager because at that point they are able to understand donor conception. But Dr. Galst says that a person's identity is largely formed by adolescence, and introducing donor conception at this time requires backtracking and correcting some of their already-formed beliefs about themselves and their family.

Expect to tell the story in different ways at different ages

Your young child is likely to enjoy the pregnancy story and have few questions about who helped you and what that help means. However, as he gets older, the story becomes more complicated. What does it mean to give "eggs"? How are these eggs different to the ones you eat for breakfast? Why did your donor help you? What does it mean to give help and receive it? And on it goes. Keep in mind what we learned from researchers at Emory about family narratives: questions about family history—and their answers—play a significant role in building self-esteem in children.

We turn to developmental psychologist Anne Bernstein for her guidance in understanding how children understand reproduction at different ages. Bernstein, who feels "What you don't know *can* hurt you" (p.30), has written a remarkable book about talking with young children about sex and reproduction. In *The Flight of the Stork: What Children Think (and When) about Sex and Family Building* (1994), she advises that when a child asks, "Where do babies come from?" a parent should first respond, "Where do you think?" This lets parent know what the child knows or guesses (p.44).

Bernstein's book guides parents through a series of six levels of cognitive development at which children understand more and more about reproduction and family connectedness. Bernstein reminds parents, again and again, that children have a great deal of curiosity about where babies come from and that talking with them at a level they can understand not only strengthens bonds between parent and child, but enhances a child's growth and development. "A child's questions about procreation are an early foray into their search for knowledge," Bernstein writes. "Encouraging the child's unguarded questions and answering responsively also encourages the child as an active, inquisitive explorer of the world" (p.29).

In *The Flight of the Stork*, Bernstein's six levels of understanding offer parents practical information about what children can understand and when they can understand it. Throughout her discussion Bernstein emphasizes the importance of parents listening very carefully to what their children are saying, reminding themselves that children really do see the world through a different lens than do adults. Bernstein also urges parents to use correct terminology about body parts. For example, it is crucial that children be told that a baby grows in a mommy's uterus or womb—not tummy—so that a child does not confuse eating or becoming full with pregnancy. Children need to know that babies have a place to grow in women—the womb or uterus. Teaching about anatomy using real names increases self-esteem and reduces confusion. And of particular significance to parents through egg donation is the need to avoid having the child confuse eggs that help create babies with those we eat for breakfast.

The following are brief summaries of each of Bernstein's (1994) levels. As we said earlier, your child will understand his story in different ways over time. You may think he "gets it" at seven and later be totally surprised by a comment he makes or a question that sounds as if it comes from a much younger child. Remember that the following levels are only guidelines, that each includes children of a rather broad age span and that the most important thing always is that you speak with confidence in your relationship with your child, regardless of his level of comprehension.

LEVEL ONE

Level one children are described by Bernstein as the "Geographers." Between ages three and seven, level one children believe that babies always existed and it is just a question of where they were before they joined their families. They learn that babies grow in their mothers' bodies, but they assume that they always existed.

Understanding level one reminds parents through egg donation that young children are not thinking about who created them and how it happened—they assume they always existed.

LEVEL TWO

Level two children are described by Bernstein as the "Manufacturers." Children reach level two between ages four and eight, and when they do, they realize that babies did not always exist; they had to be created. These manufacturers also know that a man and a woman are needed to create a baby, but they are not clear of the role each plays.

Understanding level two helps parents through egg donation introduce their role as manufacturers to their young children. They have the opportunity to let their child know that they created him together, but that others (donor, doctor) assisted them in their creation.

LEVEL THREE

Level three children are described by Bernstein as the "In-Betweens." During this transitional time, usually arrived at between ages five and ten, children explain procreation as a mixture of physiology and technology. They know Mommy and Daddy can't open and close their tummies, but they may assume that conception is impossible without marriage. At this level, they know there are three major ingredients to making babies—social relationships such as love and marriage, sexual intercourse and the union of sperm and egg—but they can't combine these factors into a coherent whole. They can be aware that their explanations don't add up.

Understanding level three assists egg donation parents as they begin to explain assisted reproduction to children. Their task is to convey to young children that sometimes love and science need to work together to create a much wanted child.

Level four

Level four children are described by Bernstein as the "Reporters." These diligent little people, between ages seven to 12, feel the most important thing is to report accurately. The world is full of laws, and they limit explanations of reproduction to the facts. They understand that paternity is not just a social relationship—it is tied to biology.

Understanding level four assists parents as they help their children grapple with the fact that someone can have a genetic connection to a child and not be a parent, and that someone can be a parent without having a genetic connection to their child.

Level five

Level five children are identified by Bernstein as the "Theoreticians." Children arrive at this level between ages ten and 13 and, in some cases, may remain there for the rest of their lives. Theoreticians see both sperm and egg as necessary, but believe that a baby really begins in one or the other.

Bernstein reminds her readers that the idea that a life began in either egg or sperm—but not both—was accepted for much of history. Only since the 1870s, she reports, have scientists realized that genetic material comes from both egg and sperm. Level five children (and adults) feel that embryos are preformed and that sexual intercourse provides conditions for them to grow.

Understanding level five can help parents of pre-teens as they put complicated pieces together, beginning to comprehend that life is created through a union of one sperm and one egg and cannot exist without both essential ingredients and the equally essential ingredient of a gestational environment.

LEVEL SIX

Level six is the point at which someone "puts it all together." According to Bernstein, level six can begin as early as 11 or 12, or it may not occur at all. Those who do reach level six "can assimilate the concept that two distinct entities, sperm and egg, can become one qualitatively different and unique entity, the embryo. Level six requires an appreciation that the genetic materials are transformed in the process of uniting" (p.145). She goes on to add that level six thinkers are ready to consider the moral and social aspects of reproduction and they "can integrate physiology with emotion, religious teaching and social convention" (p. 146).

Understanding level six helps prepare parents of donor offspring for adolescence and for the "Who am I?" questions that inevitably arise. As they watch their children grapple with the relative influences of genetics, gestation, family environment, friends, community, faith and so on, parents can feel confident in their roles and respectful of the complex questions their children are asking.

When and How will my Child Talk with Others

A question that often arises is "If I talk with my child about donor conception, he is likely to tell others. Then what do we do?" If you are asking yourself this question, you are correct: you can't talk openly and proudly with a child and then ask him not to say anything about it. That would convey quite a mixed message. Instead, we encourage you to trust that your child's conversations with others—if they occur at all—are not likely to be problematic.

"If they occur at all?" Yes, we know that children talk with their friends and their grandparents and their teachers, but they also develop a sense of privacy. Rebecca Gordon, the 11-year-old whose family was introduced in Chapter 1, has known her entire life that she was conceived through donor insemination (DI) and she was an active participant when it came time for her parents to select an egg donor. Still, Rebecca chooses not to tell her friends or teachers about her donor origins. Her parents say that they have never told her something was private—"she just knew."

This perspective is also voiced by Chicago social worker Judy Calica, who reminds us that children generally develop a clear sense of what is private in a family. Calica notes that children become attuned to social cues and advises parents to trust that their children will only talk about donor conception if and when it is appropriate.

Yes, there will be times when your child does speak about donor conception. What do you do then and what might be the consequences of these conversations?

If your child says something to others about his egg donor or about how he was born, there might be any of the following responses.

SURPRISE

If your child brings up egg donation with someone who knows what it is but didn't know that it is part of your family story, there may be a reaction of surprise. The person may be a bit confused or wonder why you didn't say something to them, but we think it is unlikely that an adult will openly convey surprise to the child. If it is someone you are close with or someone else who might have a reason to know, such as a teacher, you might hear from the person afterwards, letting you know what occurred if you were not there. If you were there, you might want to pre-empt questions by contacting the person and filling them in a bit on what you now feel they have reason to know.

CURIOSITY

Many people—including many highly educated and well-informed people—simply do not know about egg donation. They've heard of it but don't really understand what is involves medically, socially, logistically. They may have questions, possibly lots of questions. Donor egg parents report that these questions almost always seem innocent and are not judgmental. Your task, as a parent, is to respond to questions in an informative and non-defensive way while feeling the right and ability to maintain your privacy.

IT IS WHAT IT IS

On hearing that egg donation is part of your story, many people will simply respond in a neutral way. They express neither surprise nor curiosity nor judgment—theirs is simply an "it is what it is" reaction. We put in this category those who simply see egg donation as an extension of infertility treatment.

JUDGMENT/CRITICISM

We can't rule out the possibility that you will encounter a critical or judgmental response, but we think it unlikely that any criticism will be directed towards your child. If a family member or friend disapproves of egg donation, they may say something to you after hearing the news from your child. How do you deal with this? Once you get over your hurt and anger, you will remind yourself that you made your decisions with great care and that you are quite delighted with their outcome. You may then wonder what it is about your family member or friend's situation that causes them to be judgmental.

Do we really need to tell our child the truth?

Our first response to people who ask if they need to speak the truth to their child is to ask why they would consider not being truthful. Their replies usually focus on fears that the child will somehow be upset or troubled by the information that he was donor-conceived. This fear reflects the would-be parents' discomfort with egg donation and suggests that they may not be ready to move forward with the process. Counseling or perhaps discussions with other ED parents may help them feel confident and proud of their decision—or they may decide that egg donation is not for them.

It is also important to question the assumption that a child will somehow be upset or saddened by news of donor conception. Olivia Montuschi, co-founder of the Donor Conception Network in the United Kingdom and the parent of two donor-conceived young adults, offers first-hand evidence that some donor offspring feel special. She gives the example of her 25-year-old daughter,

Zannah, who likes to bring up her story in conversations if it is appropriate to do so and who has chosen to tell all her friends about her beginnings, feeling it is part of her identity. Montuschi adds that Zannah's confidence enabled her to deal with the occasional foolish comment someone made when she was younger and that, as an adult, she has never received any negative comments.

Fortunately, there is wise and informed guidance about the importance of speaking truthfully to children. This guidance comes from children of donated eggs and from donor sperm offspring who are old enough to talk about their experience.

> Daniel, 16, was conceived through egg donation. His parents have always been fully open with him and so Daniel doesn't get why people are so worried about talking with their kids. Daniel says, "It's not a big part of my life. I think it would be hard for me if I learned now that I came from a donor, but I've always known it. I'm not interested in meeting the donor, but I know that if I was, my mom would put me in the car and take me there."

The voices of donor offspring have been captured in writing and on film. In her book *Experiences of Donor Conception* (2003), Caroline Lorbach chronicles the history of secrecy in donor insemination and then tells about the pain that secrecy wrought on donor families. Lorbach offers the voices of several donor offspring, including Bill, Christine, Barry, Nicky, whom we quote below. They cover the most of the concerns of DI offspring— the value of truth telling, the avoidance of shame, the need for accurate medical information and the longing for information about the donor longing for information about the donor. While egg donation differs from sperm donation in significant ways, the words of these DI offspring seem relevant to all donor conception.

Bill tells us:

> DI parents have raised us, but, because of the shame they feel about their infertility, they are reluctant to discuss our origins with us, fearful we would reject them for their decision… They do not

understand that we are undergoing genetic bewilderment. (Lorbach 2003, p.167)

Christine, who learned the truth about her origins as an adult, says:

> I no longer have to be vigilant about the onset of the diabetes which killed my legal father and other members of his family, and I am heartily glad that I hadn't volunteered to take part in ground-breaking medical research in our locality involving people with a family history of diabetes. My involvement could have given false results and impaired the success of the whole research program. (Lorbach 2003, pp.171–172)

And from Barry:

> Things have changed, but secrecy is a legacy of that period. Secrecy is isolating; when you have a secret in the family, it is a barrier. When you have a secret, you have power over the person who does not know the secret. Many women feel the need to tell someone, and kids tend to pick up on secrets...and medically, you have to lie to a doctor when you are asked your family history. (Lorbach 2003, p.181)

And from Nicky, a more positive report:

> In my case, I have a very loving family who have done the best they could with the little they knew about donor insemination. I have always felt loved and treasured by both my mother and (social) father. They answered my questions when I sensed that Dad wasn't my biological father, and they have never resented me for or prevented me from exploring the possibility of finding out information relating to my history. I respect and thank them for that. (Lorbach 2003, pp.184–185)

Barry Stevens, also a DI offspring, has written and produced the exquisite film *Offspring* (2001). In it, Stevens chronicles the search that he and his sister undertook following the death of their father, and the news, from their mother, that they were both conceived through donor sperm. As he searches for information about his genetic father, Stevens poignantly and powerfully captures the longing of DI (and, we assume, DE) offspring to know the truth about where they came from.

Karen, a donor offspring, wrote in a personal email to me (Ellen):

> I am not adopted in the traditional sense. I know my mother, but was raised "as if" my father was actually my biological father. I wasn't told the truth until I was 16. I challenged my mother with the knowledge, and she confessed. To this day she insists that someone must have told me. No one had. It was just knowledge I had in my inner being that I blurted out one day. Anyway, to get to the point. I just attended a family reunion this weekend on my father's side of the family. I've been in a funk ever since. It is a four-and-a-half-hour drive home, and I hardly spoke the entire way and the crying started as soon as I hit home (I am a well-adjusted, functioning, member of society, 47 years old). I can only describe what I am going through as grieving. My issues seem to come in waves. First at 16, again at around 32, and now here it comes again apparently. Just when I think I have come to terms with everything, I've been blind-sided with another surge of emotions.

Blended families

Many people who turn to egg donation already have one child. Secondary infertility can occur for many reasons, but an increasingly common story is the couple who had their first child when the mom was in her late 30s or very early 40s. This first child might have arrived without difficulty or after a successful IVF cycle. Either way, they find themselves unable to have a second full genetic child and turn to egg donation. If this is your situation, inevitably, you have two central questions: "Will we have different feelings toward our children?" and "How will others react to our blended family?" We take a look here at both questions.

Will you have different feelings towards your children? Of course you will. Do you know any parent who has more than one child and can honestly say, "I feel the same feelings towards them." All of us who are blessed with two or more children can list countless ways in which our children are different from each other, and those parents who are honest with themselves and others will acknowledge that these differences trigger different feelings. The shy child may remind you of yourself as a child and you may feel extra love and compassion because you understand her so well, or frustration and even anger because you wish she could be different. You may feel closer to your son than your daughter because she is a "Daddy's little girl" and sometimes rebuffs you and he is always fiercely loyal. And on it goes.

The challenge, when you blend your family with egg donation, is to not feel unnerved by your different feelings. Your friends can grumble about how this or that child drives them crazy, while you feel you have to keep any negative reactions to your donor-conceived child in check. With donor conception as a variable, you may fear you will blame a negative feeling on the way your child joined your family.

In dealing with differences, donor parents wonder what traits came from the donor. These questions are heightened for those who never met their donor. A bothersome trait, such as stubbornness or oppositional behavior, can prompt uncomfortable feelings, especially if your genetic child has none of those traits. Sometimes the differences simply prompt curiosity, as they did with Lee, the mother of two young girls, the second born from egg donation.

"I was a tomboy," says Lee with a bit of pride. "My older daughter, Sarah, is a tomboy like me. My younger daughter, Hannah is a 'girly girly,' who loves everything pink and princess-y. I love her for all the ways she is different from me but I was curious about whether her 'girly girly-ness' is genetic. I wrote a letter to Abigail, our donor, and asked her if she loved princesses when she was a child. Abigail's response made me laugh. 'Are you kidding?' Abigail wrote. 'I was absolutely not a girly girly. I was rough and tumble and anti-pink.'" Lee smiles as she says that she was relieved to receive Abigail's response. It didn't matter to her that Hannah loves dolls and princess dress-up and everything pink. What mattered was having some handle on whether these traits had come from her donor.

Some people celebrate differences in life and others pull back from them. If you are someone who celebrates differences, the ways in which your donor-conceived child is different from others in the family may be exciting, interesting, special. If you are someone who gravitates to the familiar, differences may be harder to adjust to.

In the booklet, *Mixed Blessings* (2011), Donor Conception Network co-founder, Olivia Montuschi, writes:

> Difference does not have to be negative. Difference can be exciting, stimulating, a cause of celebration or it can be relatively neutral... something that just is...and accepted as that. Difference is only worrying or dangerous if we feel threatened by it or someone is threatening us because of it. (p.5)

How will others react to our blended family? In *Mixed Blessings*, Montuschi writes:

> It is a very good idea to share information before birth with those who matter to you in order to minimize comparisons between the siblings and with regard to who the new baby looks like. People just seem to be programmed to make these comments. It can, therefore, be helpful if those you are close to understand about the non-genetic factor. (p.7)

Many people choose donors who look like the intended mom or dad in an effort to reduce the likelihood that others will declare, "Where does she get her red curly hair from?" or "I can't believe they are sisters—they look so different." Hence, in many families, there are no dramatic differences in how the children look. However, in others, differences may be striking. For example, if your donor is a friend, you may have felt that all the wonderful things you know about her trump differences in appearance.

Back to Olivia Montuschi's observation that people "just seem to be programmed." What do you do? Our best advice is to prepare some responses to comments and questions about appearance. Here are some examples of responses to the comment "Your baby is so much darker than your older daughter":

- "She is" (and leave it at that).

- "Isn't it amazing how children come out—each so unique and special!"

- "I guess I sat in the sun more when I was pregnant."

- "Our family is made up of all shades."

Parents choose their responses depending on their mood, how they feel about the person who makes the comment, how many times the comment has already been made. The first response is simple and matter-of-fact and says a lot in a few words. The second is more elaborate but essentially conveys the same message as the first response: "If you make a dumb comment, I'll respond with something that lets you know I think the comment was dumb." The third response is playful and tries to use humor to defuse the situation. And the fourth is simply educational: ancestry is complicated and increasingly diverse, and people draw their genes from many people.

Another question that arises in blended families involves when and how to tell the older child that the younger one was donor-conceived. In some instances, the two children are very close in age and parents simply assume they will talk with both children in a natural way as they are growing up. It might go something like this with a two-year-old and a four-year-old.

"Who wants to look at pictures of when I was pregnant with each of you?" Holding the photos up, a mom might point to her belly in one photo and say, "Guess who was inside me here." Then point to the other and repeat the question. It is a happy, light-hearted encounter for two (or more) children who love hearing—yet again—the miraculous story of how they were born. Then the mom might add, "Daddy and I were so excited when I was pregnant. We couldn't wait to meet you. We wanted you each so much. We were so happy (to the younger one) that Samantha helped us with you." Neither child has any idea who Samantha is but they both hear this information—that there was a special helper the second time around.

But what happens when there are several years between the children? This often occurs with secondary infertility. Parents struggle a long time before accepting it is time to move on to egg donation. It is not far-fetched to think you will have a seven-year-old and a baby. Olivia Montuschi again offers some wise advice in this regard. She advises telling the older child early on so as to avoid having that child approach teenage years not knowing. "Teenage years are not a good age to be starting to share information of this sort and the older child might also resent not having been told earlier" (2011, p.8). She suggests talking with a child in a matter-of-fact way, noting that children don't come with the baggage of infertility and hence are unlikely to have any negative thoughts about donor conception. To those parents who express concern about respecting their younger child's privacy, Montuschi says this is unlikely to be an issue for the younger child who simply accepts his story for what it is.

Finally, there is the concern that the older child could use the information about donor conception as ammunition with the younger child. Montuschi reminds us that teasing among siblings is normal behavior and that older children sometimes try to assert their rank with their younger siblings. She doubts that older children will use information about origins to deliberately hurt a younger child but encourages parents to "keep track of what the elder child might be saying to the younger" (2011, p.8). She says that the "full implications of the non-genetic connection of their younger sibling will develop later" (2011, p.4). Montuschi advises parents to use humor to defuse potentially difficult situations and to treat remarks "lightly but authoritatively" (2011, p.8).

Relationships with donors

Donors who are family members and friends

When people decide to have a family member or friend as a donor, they usually give a great deal of thought to how the donation might affect their relationship. A common concern is that the donor will feel some parental authority and will interfere with the way the child is being raised. Fortunately, counseling and lengthy discussions between donors and their prospective recipients minimize the risk of problems. Our experience is that donors— whether they are sisters or friends or volunteer donors—really do not see themselves in a parental role.

Uninvited parental advice is but one fear that arises regarding a known donor. Another is the fear that they will feel forever indebted to the donor. After all, how can you thank someone for giving you the gift of life? As much as payment to egg donors can be troubling, it serves an important purpose: it reduces the lopsidedness of the donor–recipient relationship. For this reason, many recipients in known donation give a meaningful gift to their donors, such as a contribution to the donor's child's college fund.

Whatever feelings you have towards your donor, it will be important to accept and respect that your child will have his own feelings towards this person. For some offspring, an aunt who donated is the same aunt she would have been had she not donated. For other offspring, the relationship may feel more special because of the unique relationship that now exists between aunt and niece or nephew.

Donors whom you meet through an agency

Individuals and couples who meet their donor usually envision one meeting. Whether about to start the cycle, newly pregnant or meeting after the baby is born, the recipients want to give the donor a hug, thank her and tell her what this means to them. They also want to learn more about her and her family in an effort to have more complete information for their child. Few envision an ongoing relationship.

When they are raising a young child or children born through egg donation, some parents find that feelings change. Wendy Kramer, who heads the Donor Sibling Registry, reports that while some donors and recipients are using the DSR to remain in touch without having direct contact, more and more families are forging new forms of relationships. Kramer observes that these relationships take many forms, from those that are occasional emails to ones that celebrate and enjoy new forms of kinship. Kramer says that people sometimes say, "Well, is it like a close aunt or a godmother or…?" Kramer responds, "It really isn't like anything. It is new and unique and each situation is simply like itself." What Kramer emphasizes most is that these new relationships unfold and take different forms over time. For example…

In the two years since their twins were born, Maddy and Jack have sent occasional emails to their donor, along with photos of the twins. They were touched when their donor recently wrote to them and asked if they would be okay with her donating to another family. "We were blown away by her question. We know we have no say in whether she donates again but just the fact that she consulted us on this indicates that she feels a commitment to our family."

Another example comes with Elissa, a mom through egg donation of a three-year-old daughter, Lucy. Elissa had a wonderful pregnancy but a traumatic delivery in which she very nearly died. She recovered, both physically and emotionally, from this trauma and has spent the past three years delighting in the young daughter whom she sees as a true miracle. Recently, she felt a desire to share some of what she had been through with her donor:

> I sat down and wrote her a ten-page letter telling her everything. I told her what I went through in childbirth and I wrote a lot about my fantastic little girl. I took ample opportunity to thank her. I was so happy when she wrote back. It was the most wonderful and understanding letter! She said great things about Lucy and she was so kind and compassionate about my hysterectomy. She wrote me a lot about herself and her family. Reading her letter made me so happy. It made me so excited about Lucy meeting her one day.

Donors who remain anonymous

Among the lessons adult DI offspring have offered us is that many children conceived through donor gametes have a deep and often abiding curiosity about their donor. Their feelings are very similar to those reported by generations of adult adoptees, their parents and birth parents—feelings that have greatly influenced the growing trend toward more openness in adoption. This curiosity is one of the reasons why recipients of anonymous donation try to obtain as much information as possible about their donor. While you are raising your child, you are likely to find that the donor comes and goes from your mind.

Your child, also, is likely to have intermittent thoughts and feelings about the donor. In the absence of information, he/she may have fantasies. We hope you will have information about the donor that will help your child sort through some of these fantasies. For example, a photo will help your daughter if she is wondering if the donor is someone she saw at the mall or on TV. Photos of her family and the questionnaire she filled out will also be important to your child. Sometimes recipients request and get additional information that they save for the child. I (Ellen) know a couple who composed several questions for their donor and asked the agency to videotape her replying to them. That video is something they are happy to have for their child.

Information about the donor's family and about the other families she donated to will help your son who wonders if his new girlfriend could be genetically related to him. Adoptees and DI offspring have taught us that children have these fantasies and questions, that they somehow cope with them and that the most important thing for parents to do is to continue to talk openly and honestly with their children. Remember that your children can accept the fact that you have limited information as long as they know that they can count on you to speak with them with sincerity and compassion. If they become angry with you, try not to become defensive or apologetic. You did the best you could when you chose egg donation, and now you are doing the best you can to raise your child with the information that is available to you.

Remember that things sometimes change. You may not know your donor now but you may find a way of connecting with her sometime in the future.

Feelings common to many parents after infertility

As we said at the start of this chapter, our focus here is on issues that might arise for parents through egg donation. We turn our attention here to feelings that are often experienced by parents through egg donation as well as other parents after infertility.

The obligation to be eternally grateful

When they are going through infertility treatment, people make bargains. Among them is the pledge "If only I am able to have a baby, I will be eternally grateful." When a real live child comes along, parents are grateful—very grateful—but they are also tired, stressed, ambivalent and inexperienced. It is difficult to maintain a consistently high level of gratitude, but that is what they feel they have pledged to do. Many become angry with themselves and remorseful when they feel the normal feelings of new parents—fatigue, trapped and wondering, "What have I gotten myself into?"

Parents who feel committed to eternal gratitude may find it more difficult to discipline their children. You know that your child needs limits, but you may feel as if you are being cruel and ungrateful if you say "no" to him. Logically, this makes no sense but there is a lot of illogical thinking connected to infertility and parenting after infertility. Having endured so much disappointment and loss, parents sometimes associate leniency with gratitude—"If I love him so much and am so grateful to have him, then how can I punish him?"

Questions of authenticity

"What do you know about her real mother?" This question has plagued adoptive mothers for years and it can undermine moms through egg donation as well. Pregnancy is authenticating, and labor and delivery can surely seal the deal. Once they have brought a child into the world, ED moms feel pretty certain that they are the "real thing." But certainly in the beginning, feelings of being a fake or a fraud or "found out" are torturous. Again, we blame those who suggest that there is something to keep a secret about and who talk about "disclosure."

Feelings about being older parents

Parents through egg donation are often older parents, either because they first attempted parenthood at advanced age or because they spent years pursuing pregnancy on their own or years considering and pursuing egg donation.

Whatever got them to advanced age, all older parents face certain issues. One is the fact that their own parents are older, or, perhaps, have died along the way. There is a loss of grandparenting, or, for some, there is the experience of being in "the sandwich generation"—having to meet the needs of young children and aging parents at the same time.

There are also worries about their own age and health. Many illnesses and medical conditions become more common when people are in their 40s. New parents may be surprised by how tired they are taking care of a baby and begin to worry about what it will be like in a few years, let alone when their child reaches adolescence.

Questions of family planning

Among the many legacies of infertility is the inability to plan your family. While your fertile friends are busy talking about timing and ideal spacing, you may be wondering whether you will be able to afford another donor cycle. Or perhaps you are worrying about your cryopreserved embryos or thinking a lot about whether you can ask your sister or close friend to donate again. You may also be focusing on your age, feeling that you cannot delay adding to your family because you don't want to be any older when your next child is born.

How nice it would be to enjoy your long-awaited first child and wait a year or two or three before adding to your family. Unfortunately, the concerns we just listed and the inevitable fear that it will take a long time to achieve another pregnancy prevent many parents though egg donation from postponing decisions about adding to their family. Those who want to remain a one-child family and those who have twins and feel their family is complete are spared family planning worries, but most others are not.

Feeling caught between the fertile and infertile worlds

In the fertile world, women can talk endlessly about pregnancy, labor and delivery. They can moan about stretch marks or groan that they had a C-section. Now you are among them, but your experience may seem vastly different. You may have labored for years to have a baby and a few extra hours in labor are of little consequence. Yes, you are having some trouble taking off the weight you gained, but you don't mind it all that much—it's a temporary souvenir of your pregnancy.

So one way that you are caught between the fertile and infertile worlds is that you are with fertile moms and you feel different. Another place you feel different is with infertile women—you may feel that you are still one of them, but sometimes they don't see it that way. You have had a baby and that puts you in a new place.

Although it is important for you to be with other moms— "regular" other moms—you will probably also find it helpful to connect with other moms through egg donation. If you are in the US, you should be able to access them through your local RESOLVE or AFA, or through Parents Via Egg Donation (PVED), which offers a blog, forums and other helpful ways of connecting with other donor parents. The Donor Conception

Network in the UK offers workshops, conferences, and advocacy as well as social and informal parent and family gatherings. In Israel there is Israel Donor Families, in Canada, the Infertility Network, The Australian Donor Conception Network offers social events in major Australian cities and the list goes on. We hope you get the point—there are lots of ways of connecting with other donor families.

Our real vs. our fantasy children

When contemplating parenthood, everyone fantasizes about what their child will be like. Inevitably, partners focus on the traits they like best in themselves and in each other, and they imagine a child who combines the best of both of them. In anticipating parenthood, it is much easier and more natural to picture a child with her beautiful eyes and his great hair or her athletic ability and his musical talent than it is to imagine a child who has her anxiety and his stubbornness, her Uncle Fred's schizophrenia genes and his Aunt Sally's paranoia. You get the picture.

Our real children are not the children of our fantasies. They are not exactly who we expected, but, as parents, we realize that our task is to love them for who they are and not for who they are not. This can be a challenge for all parents, but perhaps all the more so for donor conception parents. While other parents can celebrate differences with a sense of curiosity and wonder, you may be more inclined to experience disappointment. If you had an anonymous donor, you may be wondering whether your child has inherited some of his less appealing traits from the donor. You may feel added sadness that some qualities you'd hoped to see in your child seem to be missing.

We encourage parents through egg donation to realize that all parents deal with disappointment. As much as we love our children, they are always different in some way from what we wanted and hoped they would be. And that, in many ways, is the magic of parenthood. Philosophy professor Michael J. Sandel concludes his article, "The case against perfection" (2004) with these words about those who seek to "design" children: "But that promise of mastery is flawed. It threatens to banish our appreciation of life as a gift and to leave us with nothing to affirm or behold outside our own will."

Extraordinary joy

Lest we end on a down note, we turn now to the most prominent feature of parenting after infertility: JOY. Ecstasy. Exuberance.

How often we have seen people who struggled and struggled to build their family be transformed into content and happy parents. Yes, they are tired. Sure, they feel ambivalence. But what we notice most of all is their happiness. They look younger, they look more relaxed; their cars and their homes and their very selves are permanently altered.

In her wise and comforting essay "Entitled to all that parenting has to offer" (2008) psychologist Carole Lieber Wilkins, herself a mom through egg donation and adoption, concludes with these words:

> We get it all. Whether infertile or not, genetically related or not, whether we gave birth to them or not, we are entitled to all the title of Mom and Dad confers upon us—the blessing and the curse— with our eyes open and fully cognizant of the blessing which we have finally received.

– 9 –

Ethics and Faith

Egg donation is very much a journey of the heart. Throughout this book we have tried to approach your journey through an ethical perspective. We turn now to a more comprehensive overview of medical ethics as they relate to egg donation and to matters of faith and belief.

An overview of ethics

Ethics are a set of principles that motivate us to engage in morally right behavior. Each of us has our own unique personal code of ethics and specific definitions of behaviors we feel are right and wrong. Our personal code of ethics has been developed and influenced by many factors in our lives—our family culture, our religious training, our schooling and so on. We draw upon this code of ethics when we need to make difficult decisions. For most of us, it is our ethics that we rely upon to guide us and keep us from crossing ethical lines in situations that may tempt us. The use of donated eggs to form families is complex ethically because it raises many questions that we never thought we would have to think about, and it forces us to carefully consider new ways of creating families.

Ethics related to medical and health issues are governed by four major principles. The first is autonomy—the obligation to respect the decision-making rights of individual people. This allows each individual patient to decide which course of treatment to pursue or refuse. Regardless of how strong your views are, however, it is difficult to predict what you will do in a situation until you are actually faced with it. It is the responsibility of medical professionals to ensure that each patient is accurately informed about his medical condition and all of the treatment possibilities that are available, and then to respect that each patient has the autonomy to make his decision on his own. As long as it does not infringe on the welfare and safety of others, autonomy encourages us to assume that everyone is making the best decision possible for themselves and their families.

The next two principles—non-maleficence and beneficence—go hand in hand. Non-maleficence emphasizes the obligation to "do no harm," while beneficence encourages not only the obligation to actually provide benefits but also to balance these benefits against risks. With egg donation, it is easy to see that a benefit would be that a couple gets a new baby, but is there the potential of harm to the donor, the baby or even the joyful new parents? In examining the potential for harm in egg donation, issues surrounding anonymity, payment, medical and psychological risks to the donor and the feelings of her extended family all need to be acknowledged. The bottom line is that we do not know the long-term effects of egg donation.

The final medical health ethical principle is justice. Justice obligates fairness in the distribution of benefits and risks. In other words, everyone should be treated fairly and have access to what they need, including the most advanced forms of reproductive technology. While most of us would agree with this concept in theory, the reality is much more complicated. Since reproductive technologies are not typically covered by insurance nor are they available in every small town, there are limits as to who has access to these technologies and who does not. This raises the question of who should control these limits and ultimately decide who should be able to attempt certain ARTs and collaborative reproductive options, including egg donation. Often, it is money that speaks the loudest. Is it fair to assume that just because you have enough money to spend, you have the right to attempt to conceive with donated eggs despite the circumstances?

When any of these principles clash, an ethical dilemma results, and we are forced to ask the age-old question: "Just because we can do it, should we?" Since autonomy is the cornerstone of medical ethics, in most instances medical professionals are inclined to accept a patient's autonomy and respect her right to make any decisions that she feels are in her best interests. However, is it always acceptable to allow someone to do this, especially when it may cause possible harm in the future, as perhaps may be the case with egg donation? Moreover, who should have the power to make these "gate-keeping" decisions?

Your ethical decision making

As with most ethical questions, there are very few absolute right or wrong answers here. As we have said before, you will encounter many different opinions and point of views over the course of your journey, from family and friends as well as respected professionals such as clergy and physicians. They will all claim that they are indeed right regarding their views on egg donation. Consequently, this experience will challenge you to rely on your own ethical and moral frameworks to navigate through these gray areas. Our goal for this chapter is to better prepare you to face these difficult issues with knowledge and confidence as you travel down the road toward egg donation. We sincerely hope that you take from this book as much information as possible and decide what is best for you and your family, while taking into careful consideration all the risks and benefits and the overall justice of your final decision.

The evolution of egg donation

More than 30 years ago, when IVF was in its infancy, it was almost immediately met with worldwide public outcry. Most of Western civilization felt that assisted reproductive technology was "against God's will" and feared that it would destroy traditional family values that had long been established and actively promoted within society. Physicians and scientists throughout the world argued about the ethics of IVF and its implications. With one in seven couples unable to conceive on their own, supporters of IVF thought it a valid means to help many couples realize their dream of becoming pregnant. How could they deny couples this chance—most likely their only chance—to have a baby? On the other hand, there were many who thought IVF was just one step further down a slippery slope. "What is so slippery about giving people the chance to have babies?" you may ask yourself. It is important to remember that many consider IVF as the first step towards genetic engineering, creating "designer" babies and perhaps new species, as well as stem cell research and cloning, all of which remain political hotbeds even as we write. In the words of Eunice Kennedy Shriver, "Even beneficial developments can be the first step on a slope that might lead to great harm."

Where are we today? Some counties, such as Austria, Norway, Sweden and Switzerland, have completely banned the use of donated eggs, mainly due to the slippery-slope philosophy, having decided that the benefits just do not outweigh the risks involved. Other counties, such as the United Kingdom, Australia and Canada, have put in place specific regulations concerning use of donated eggs in the hope of mitigating these risks. In the United States, thousands of babies have been born through the use of egg donation. Even though there will always be some who oppose assisted reproduction in almost all cases or more specifically gamete donation or other third-party reproduction, egg donation, generally speaking, has come to be accepted by American society as an appropriate means to build a family.

However, we still have not found the answers to so many of the major ethical questions raised by egg donation, such as "When do we cross the line and cause harm?" It seems as though the obvious benefits of reproductive technology are surpassing our ability to fully comprehend and reconcile concerns we might have. To make matters worse, no one can decide who should further explore these issues. Many governments, including the United States government, have been reluctant to take a stance on egg donation—specifically, about what should be allowed and what should not. This puts anyone who is considering using donated eggs in a difficult place. How can you be expected to make important life-altering decisions about egg donation when so many others, including prominent leaders across various disciplines such as medicine, science, theology and law, who deal with similar tough ethical issues every day, have not been able to do so?

Now back to the original question: is egg donation ethical? We believe that there are ethically sound ways to become parents through egg donation but acknowledge that not everyone feels this way. Your decision is yours to make and should be based on your own sense of personal ethics. What is right for someone else may not be right for you, and vice versa. It is our hope that this chapter will provide you with the knowledge and tools to guide you and help you feel good about making vital decisions that will affect you and your family and a potential donor and her family for the rest of your lives.

In whose best interest?

In order for egg donation to be ethically sound, all participants should enjoy some benefit or beneficence. Their autonomy should be respected and they should be treated with justice. By "all," we refer to the offspring, the recipients, members of their extended families and society at large. Let's take a look at what might be in the best interests of each group.

The offspring

We begin with the question of the best interests of the children since, unlike the donors and recipients, the offspring of donated eggs cannot speak for themselves—at least not at the time of key decision making. Who, then, looks after their best interests and what might these interests involve?

On the positive side, children created through egg donation are given the gift of life, something they would not otherwise have and the value of which may trump any negatives associated with egg donation. Add to the gift of life the fact that these are children who are wanted, planned for and will be raised by those who intended, from the start, to parent them.

If children created using donated eggs are given gifts of life, love and family, then surely it can be argued that egg donation is ethically sound. However, that does not negate the losses experienced by some egg donation offspring. There are those who are permanently cut off from one side of their genetic families. This occurs not only because some donors remain anonymous but also because some donors donate multiple times. The Donor Sibling Registry (DSR) has made it much easier for donor offspring to find or identify one another, but vast numbers of donor offspring are not part of the DSR.

Although egg donation is fundamentally different from sperm donation, since egg donors undergo significant inconvenience, discomfort and even risk to donate, it is possible that some offspring will react in much the same way as those sperm donor offspring who accuse their donor fathers of "doing it for the money."

Cultural differences impact the experiences of offspring. While some countries, including the UK, Finland, Norway, Holland, Switzerland, Austria, Germany, New Zealand, and four states in Australia, now ban anonymous donation. In other countries, such as Israel, anonymity prevails. In her article, "In Search of Donor Relations and Identity: The Missing Voices of Israel's Children," Dr. Ruth Shidlo cites the 1989 UN Convention on the Rights of the Child and questions whether Israel's laws, preserving anonymity, "constitute 'lawful interference' with the offspring's right to preserve his or her identity and establish family relations with the donor parent and/or siblings" (Shidlo 2012, p.648).

Some donor offspring will be born to older parents, and this raises further questions about what is in their best interests. Although it was always possible for a child to be born to a 60-year-old man, prior to the availability of egg donation the mother was almost always under 45. It is now possible for a child to be born to two people over 45 or even significantly older. Is it in a child's best interests to have parents who are over 60 when raising an adolescent? Is egg donation creating children who will need to take care of elderly parents before they themselves really reach adulthood? Does it create children whose parents are likely to die before they themselves have gotten through an increasingly lengthening adolescence (now presumed to include not just the teen years, but also a significant portion of the 20s)?

In her article, "How older parenthood will upend American society: the scary consequences of the grayest generation" (Shulevitz 2012b), journalist Judith Shulevitz, who became a mother at 39 raises many concerns about older parenthood. These include a higher risk for learning problems, attention deficit disorders, autism, etc. Shulevitz also writes about what it means for people to have fewer children than they would have otherwise wanted as well as the potential for loss of the important grandparent-grandchild relationship. She notes that in addition to offering all sorts of support to younger parents, grandparents have traditionally forged special bonds with their grandchildren and they have been the bearers of family traditions. Shulevitz observes that if her son waits until age 39 to have his first child, she will become a grandmother at nearly 80, an age at which many people are no longer able to play actively and energetically with young children.

And so we see, in reviewing ethical principles, that, when it comes to donor offspring, some fundamental questions arise. Surely the gifts of life, love and family are evidence of beneficence, but when we look at the potential suffering associated with being cut off from genetic relatives and history and being born to older parents, we see that, for some egg donation offspring, there are questions of justice and non-maleficence.

The donors

Does egg donation offer benefit to donors? Where do the other central ethical principles of autonomy and justice fit in? From a positive perspective, egg donation respects a donor's autonomy. A woman can decide to donate her eggs to her sister in need, to a close friend, or she can become an altruistic donor.

Researcher Judith Bernstein documented in Seibel and Crockin's book *Family Building through Egg and Sperm Donation: Medical, Legal and Ethical Issues* (1996) and others have observed that egg donation offers donors "gratification through altruism, increased self-esteem or fulfillment of a desire to rework a negative past experience with a better outcome" (p.332). At the same time, however, Judith Bernstein and others address the question of non-maleficence—the potential for a donor to be vulnerable to harm, either psychological or physical, as a result of the donation. Harm could occur if a family member feels coerced into donating, if a volunteer donor is enticed by payment or if a medical or egg donation program does not go to great lengths to help donors achieve informed consent.

EDUCATION AND INFORMATION SHARING
With true informed consent, women donating eggs would be likely to recognize their need to know the outcome of their donation. They would understand that if their efforts to help a family have a child are successful, that child may want to know more about the person who helped give him life. The truly informed donor would be prepared for a future in which questions might arise, coming either from the offspring or the recipient, or they may arise within the donor herself. Unfortunately, true informed consent does not always occur. There are donors who are left wondering what happened with their eggs and if there is "a piece of me out there" and who are, indeed, harmed by the process. According to one study conducted by the Bioethics Institute at the Johns Hopkins University (Kalfoglou and Geller 2000), most egg donors interviewed after their donations would, in retrospect, like to have known what happened to their donated eggs. The most common reason for this was that it would make them feel good to know that their donation was successful.

As with any medical procedure, there is also the potential for medical complications for the egg donor. The 2011 documentary *Eggsploitation*, produced by the Center for Bioethics and Culture, raises the alarm regarding medical complications. The film chronicles the medical problems faced post-donation by a group of young women. Although it is not clear that all of their problems were the result of their donor cycle, the film raises important issues. Powerful fertility medications are used, as well as complicated surgical procedures. This raises the potential for physical risks, both short- and long-term. For example, there are risks to the donor of ovarian hyperstimulation, infection during egg retrieval, the potential for future infertility issues of her own and the possibility of increased risks for certain types of cancers, including ovarian cancer. The question arises as to whether it is beneficent to encourage healthy women to undergo ovarian hyperstimulation and egg retrieval in order to assist others to create a baby and how much information they should receive about these potential risks.

Lack of long-term follow-up among egg donors is also an ethical concern. While many clinics are now doing more to maintain contact with previous donors, for the most part, once the egg donor has donated her eggs, she is released with no further contact or follow-up. As we have mentioned, maintaining contact with egg donors is important for several reasons. First, if any of the donor's health information changes (which is quite probable given the young age of donors), it is important for her to let the clinic know so they can let the recipient family know. Second, if a donor experiences any complications that may relate to her egg donation, it is important to record this in order to ensure the safety of the egg donation process. Right now, this is not tracked at all. Another issue involves information sharing with the donor's family. In "Not in Front of the Children," Dr. Gillian Lockwood of Midland Fertility Services raises concerns for the donors of other children, current and future. In many instances, they may never be told they have "half siblings" and even those who know that their mother was a donor, are unlikely to know how many "half-sibs" they have, who and where they are.

Wendy Kramer, together with Drs. Jennifer Schneider and Natalie Schultz, contacted 287 egg donors following their donations and report their findings in their 2009 article in

Human Reproduction entitled "US oocyte donors: a retrospective study of medical and psychosocial issues." The authors received responses from 155 donors. The article raises many concerns but focuses primarily on the lack of follow-up with donors. Sadly, only 2.6 percent of the women said they had ever been contacted for follow-up by the clinic. However, over one-third reported medical changes that they thought would interest donor offspring. The researchers note that only half of these women tried to contact their clinics to let them know about the medical changes, which included infertility, ovarian hyperstimulation and menstrual changes. They reported mixed experiences talking with their clinics. Those that did not contact their clinics said they did not know they should do so.

Similarly, Dr. Jennifer Schneider wrote an article in 2008 entitled "Fatal colon cancer in a young egg donor: a physician mother's call for follow-up and research on the long-term risks of ovarian hyperstimulation." Because her daughter developed a rare and fatal type of colon cancer at such a young age, Schneider wonders if this could be somehow connected to her egg donation. Due to the lack of follow-up among egg donor programs, there is no way to gather information that would either support or reject this connection.

Conflicts of interest

Protecting donors from risks is more complicated than it seems. In their article "Navigating conflict of interest in oocyte donation: an analysis of donors' experiences" (2000), Andrea Kalfoglou, and Gail Geller, both of the Bioethics Institute at the Johns Hopkins University, explore the issue that egg donation places egg donors in a unique situation. Egg donors are not truly patients. They are not seeking medical attention in order to achieve better health. Instead, they are perfectly healthy individuals who are volunteering to undergo medical procedures that are being paid for privately by someone else to help the recipient (often someone they do not even know, in the case of anonymous donation) have a baby.

Kalfoglou and Geller raise many questions. First, what exactly is the role of the egg donor and what are the recipients' and the medical community's expectations of and responsibilities towards her? For example, when she undergoes psychological screening to be an egg donor, whose interest is the mental health professional looking out for—hers or the recipient couple's? In their study about donors' experiences, Kalfaglou and Geller illustrate this point through a quote by egg donor Claire, age unknown, who commented without any prompting:

> I was sort of curious to see how [the mental health counselor] handled her position in terms of disclosure and that sort of thing— about what her purpose was. And I expected her to say, "I am being paid by the recipient couple. I am not your advocate." Nothing. She did not even have me sign a release, which I thought was a little tacky. (2000, p.664)

Kalfoglou and Geller point out that mental health professionals' ability to provide appropriate care may be clouded by the fact that it is the recipient who is paying the entire bill and it is the recipient who wants to find an egg donor. Hence, the mental health professional may feel pressure, whether overt or more subtle, to secure a good egg donor candidate for this couple. Similarly, because the prospective donor knows the mental health professionals want to find someone who is emotionally stable and free from mental illness, she might be reluctant to provide any information—such as abuse, rape or abortion—that might put her in a bad light or hurt her chances of becoming a donor.

Another issue that arises involves the "reserving" of donors one or two cycles in advance. Some egg donor agencies will allow— even encourage—intended parents to "book" a donor for a future cycle while she is in the midst of the egg donation process. If the idea with egg donation is that a woman is electing to help a specific individual or couple build their family—even if she does not know them—shouldn't the decision to help another family be made free and clear of the first decision? What if she donates and does not want to do so again for whatever reason? What if she wants to donate once more but only to the family she has already helped? Does "reserving" her in advance not compromise her autonomy?

Likewise, conflict of interest and poorly defined roles may affect the donor's treatment by medical and legal professionals as well. Again, it is the recipient couple, not her, who pays the bills for the medical treatment and any legal representation. Consequently, donors may be unclear about their own rights and responsibilities when they agree to treatment or sign contracts. Because people are taught to trust people in authority positions, including doctors and lawyers, donors may be more hesitant to ask questions and voice concerns. Whose interest is actually being protected during the egg donation process—that of the recipient couple who is paying the clinic, lawyers and psychologists for services, or the donor who is being evaluated and screened?

COMPENSATION

Payment to donors has long been the subject of extensive ethical debate. On the one hand, compensation for time and effort and the inclusion of a broad range of women as donors meets the ethical standard of justice. The process is time-consuming, intrusive, invasive and carries with it risks, so why shouldn't women receive compensation for their effort? However, some wonder whether payments do not serve to entice women who might not otherwise donate eggs. In her essay "What Is Wrong with Commodification?" (1996, pp.106–121), Ruth Macklin, Professor of Bioethics at Albert Einstein Medical College, examines the question of payment to donors from a variety of ethical perspectives. She concludes that it all comes down to a "disagreement over commodification." Macklin explains that those who favor payment argue that to prohibit payment would be "moralistic and symbolic" (ibid) while those who oppose it say that it treats reproductive capacity as "just another market force and leads to 'an inferior conception of human flourishing'"(ibid). Macklin herself concludes that "although commodification is not immoral, it is nonetheless 'unsavory'"(ibid).

Popular media has indicated that egg donation is a booming multi-million dollar business, and desirable women are being coerced, often receiving in excess of $100,000 for their eggs. Some women have publicly recounted their horror stories of donating eggs in "greedy" egg donor programs and to desperate intended parents going to extreme lengths to secure egg donors. In 2007 The American Society for Reproductive Medicine issued guidelines regarding egg donation that attempted to offer some protection for egg donors. They recommended that women donate no more than a total of six times and stated that compensations "be based in a reasonable assessment of the time, inconvenience and discomfort associated with egg retrieval" (pp.307–308). ASRM suggested that this compensation between $5000 and $8000 and not exceed $10,000. In addition, recommendations were made to physicians to treat egg donors as they would other patients, noting burdens and risks when they advertise for egg donors.

However, it is important to know that there are no repercussions for not following these guidelines. Under this type of self-regulation policy, many clinics and donor programs are ultimately allowed to make their own decisions as how to best compete in the marketplace and satisfy their particular clients. While most clinics are respectful of ASRM's recommendations, it is naïve to think that this is always the case.

Dr. Aaron Levine of the School of Public Policy at the Georgia Institute of Technology has conducted several studies (2010a and b) looking at the oversight and practice of egg donation in the United States and abroad. There is no doubt that the current supply of egg donors does not meet the demand. To attract more potential donors, some programs use compensation as an incentive, and this has increased over time. While egg donor compensation started at about $900 to $1200 in the late 1980s, Levine found that nearly half of all egg donor advertisements placed in college newspapers today offered compensation exceeding the recommended levels set by ASRM. According to Levine, a legal limit on compensation would eliminate the worst of the abuses. At the very least, ASRM might want to take steps to improve compliance with current guidelines. On the other hand, other experts, especially those in the United Kingdom and Canada where donor compensation is prohibited, suggest that properly constructed donor programs could be successful in recruiting a good supply of altruistic donors by providing them with the respect and positive affirmation they deserve. Critics of completely altruistic donation warn that lack of compensation would severely limit the number of available donors. This is a difficult dilemma and not one that is likely to be solved anytime soon.

A related question that many grapple with is whether it is ethical to buy and sell human eggs if it is illegal to sell human organs. As we have said many times, those involved in egg donation are always careful to identify the payment as being one for time and effort, rather than for eggs. Still, the debate continues as to how like and different eggs are from human organs. Blood and bone marrow have a history of being donated for money. However, unlike egg donation, blood, bone marrow and even sperm are all replenishable and have low or no risks involved. As a result, they bring relatively low payments. In her article "What Is Wrong with Commodification?" (1996), Macklin points out that "even the sale of blood, like other human bodily materials, is a form of commodification" (p.110). Macklin quotes the Glover Report to the European Commission (1989) by Jonathan Glover and others, which observes that payment "deprives donors of the chance of doing something purely for others" (ibid).

In today's environment, Attorney Crockin recommends that intended parents can ensure that egg donation remains ethical and is not identified as the "buying and selling of eggs" by working legally within the system and having payments to donors that clearly reflect the expense, inconvenience, time involved and, according to ASRM guidelines, to some degree the risk and discomfort undertaken. Payments are typically structured over the course of a donor's efforts. Moreover, payments should not be linked to specific characteristics or outcomes, meaning egg donors that are compensated for their time and effort regardless of what happens in terms of the number of eggs retrieved, eggs fertilized or successful pregnancies or births. Nor should "proven donors"—ones who have successfully completed one or more cycles—receive higher fees than first time donors.

So what does this mean for women who volunteer to be egg donors and receive payment for doing so? For some, not much at all: they work hard to donate their eggs and are grateful to have some financial compensation for loss of work, social and leisure time. For others, however, there may be the potential for future regret. Should these women face infertility or pregnancy loss in the future, we hope that they will not look back with regret, a regret that could be intensified if the payment was at all a factor in their decision making.

Egg sharing

We turn now to egg-sharing donors. Egg sharing asks a woman who is undergoing infertility treatments to donate some of her eggs in exchange for a reduction in the costs of her treatment. Egg sharing is especially common in the UK and in Israel.

Egg sharing raises substantial ethical concerns. We all know how much infertile women long to become pregnant and the lengths many will go to to have a child. A women who can afford treatment only by giving some of her eggs to another woman could seem to be in an untenable situation. However, the April 23, 2012, edition of *BioNews* presents some interesting research on egg sharing. In her article "Evaluating egg-sharing: new findings on old debates," Dr. Zeynep Gurtin-Broadbent reports research conducted by herself and Professor Susan Golombok at the University of Cambridge Centre for Family Research. Their two-year study offered several interesting findings regarding egg sharing.

They found no significant differences in terms of the demographics of donors and recipients in egg sharing, with women coming from similar backgrounds in terms of religion, ethnicity and education. Not surprisingly, donors were on average 11 years younger than recipients (33 compared to 44 years old). The researchers looked at how the donors and recipients viewed egg sharing in terms of informed consent and exploitation and found that 88 percent of the donors and 76 percent of the recipients disagreed with the statement "egg sharing is exploitative." The large majority of donors (87%) were glad to have taken part in egg sharing and would do it again. In addition, they found that there was openness between donors and recipients, goodwill and a strong sense of reciprocity and empathy. When women were asked to describe their feelings towards their egg-sharing partner, the most common responses were curiosity (71% of donors and 78% of recipients) and hope that the other woman's treatment was successful (79% of donors and 86% of recipients). The researchers also found that unsuccessful egg share donors were no different from successful donors with regard to how often they thought about any children the recipient conceived and on feelings about possible future contact.

Olivia Montuschi, co-founder of the Donor Conception (DC) Network in the UK, says that this research supports what she has seen through the DC Network, which supports egg sharing, seeing it as in the best interests of children. She notes that if women did not share eggs, more women would travel for affordable egg donation to countries where donors were anonymous. Montuschi writes:

> Egg sharing is sometimes treated as the less acceptable face of gamete donation. Egg sharing is a scheme by which a woman under 35 who is already undergoing IVF, agrees to share the "crop" of eggs she produces with another woman who, for a range of reasons, does not have eggs that can produce a viable pregnancy. This happens in exchange for free or subsidized fertility treatment for the donor. An immediate response to this might be that the practice is exploitative, taking advantage of women at a particularly vulnerable time, both emotionally and financially. And what if the recipient becomes pregnant but the donor doesn't?
>
> Isn't this going to cause psychological damage for unsuccessful donors who will be traumatized by thoughts of the recipient conceiving their genetic children?
>
> All the above are very proper fears and anxieties, but recent research seems to be confirming anecdotal evidence that has been

leaking out for years: that empathy and a sense of reciprocity between the women involved can make egg sharing a win/win situation for both families. Women also talk about the importance of being able to help someone else have a baby—completely understanding the pain of infertility for themselves.

Obviously, there need to be very clear and fair protocols in clinics. Donors must be women whose egg quality is not compromised, so they are likely to be having IVF because of blocked fallopian tubes or for male factor reasons. There must be agreements about how the eggs are to be shared and what happens if too few eggs are produced to give each a reasonable chance. And, of course, both parties must have good pre-treatment counseling to make sure that the long-term implications of the transaction are understood and accepted. Another factor to take into account is that, in egg sharing, the donor would be undergoing artificial stimulation of egg production anyway for her own benefit. In some countries, notably pro-natalist Israel, egg sharing is the only form of egg donation allowed, it being considered unethical to stimulate a woman who is not in need of fertility treatment herself. (Montuschi 2012)

The July 7, 2012, issue of the *The Guardian* included an article about a couple, Suzanne and Mark Harper, who had a child through sperm donation and who decided, when trying for a second child, to participate in egg sharing (Moorhead 2012). Suzanne said that she was so grateful to have a child that it made her feel good to be able to help others. As it turned out, she did not conceive but the recipient did. The clinic told Suzanne that it was a twin pregnancy and it was going well. Suzanne said that she never felt envious, even when she tried again with a frozen embryo transfer and had a miscarriage. Instead, she said, "I'll always cherish the knowledge that somewhere out there there's another family who only happened because of our heartache."

The article goes on to talk about how Suzanne and Mark's experience with an anonymous sperm donor prompted them to share as much information as possible with the recipient of her eggs.

The recipients

For the recipients of donated eggs, there appear to be many advantages to receiving donated eggs, and the process seems to meet ethical measures of autonomy in that people who seek parenthood have an opportunity to make decisions for themselves; justice in that egg donation is available to a vast range of would-be parents; non-maleficence since, as long as donors have informed consent, there appears to be no harm; and beneficence, because, as we have said many times, the child created through egg donation is planned for, wanted and deeply loved. All of this is true, but there are other perspectives that can be applied to the question "Is egg donation in the best interests of the recipients?"

Some people feel a need to try to conceive using donated eggs, despite its emotional and physical risks, "because it is there." Some say that their medical programs promote egg donation as a form of treatment, rather than correctly identifying it as an alternative path to parenthood. These patients say that adoption is presented as much more challenging, risky and unfamiliar. In addition, there are instances in states with insurance mandates where egg donation is presented as much more affordable. This occurs often in Massachusetts, where there has been an insurance mandate to cover ARTs since 1987. As a result, I (Ellen) have seen a vast number of couples who have said that, without the mandate, they would have adopted, but adoption often costs close to $30,000 (now reduced by the tax credit and other adoption benefits) while egg donation could cost as little as $6000 (if the donor is a family member and medical costs are covered, there are only legal and counseling fees remaining).

Those who pursue egg donation "because it is there" and successfully become pregnant may suffer some harm because they have a child they may not be fully prepared to welcome into their families. Those who do not conceive are likely to suffer greater maleficence—egg donation becomes another failure, another setback, and for those who would otherwise chose adoption, it costs them valuable time and money.

Another aspect of the "because it is there" perspective on egg donation is that there will be recipients who pursue conception through egg donation at advanced age. At one time, women past their early 40s made peace with the fact that they could not bear children and faced big challenges adopting (challenges that have diminished greatly as some are adopting even into their 50s). Now this cohort of women has the opportunity to become pregnant, and some feel that if the opportunity is there, they should seize it. I (Ellen) recently met with a 47-year-old, newly married woman who raised serious concerns about whether it was "right for me to have a baby at this age," but who felt she should try it because "I would love to be pregnant and the doctors say it can happen."

It can happen, but is it in the best interests of recipient couples to enter into parenthood if both are of advanced age? We realize, of course, that there are 43-year-old women with 33-year-old husbands now becoming families through egg donation, but what of the couple in which both are past 45? As one medical program I (Ellen) worked in determined it, "It does not seem right to us to work with couples whose combined age is over 90." At some clinics, however, such couples are becoming parents and their advanced age may put a burden not only on their children but on the couple as well. A friend who is an elementary school principal observed, "People in their 50s with kids in elementary school are out of the loop of the parent network. They stand out as different and receive limited support from the community at a time when they could use it most." Another friend, a radiologist specializing in breast disease, said:

> Every day I have to talk with women in their 40s and 50s about a new breast cancer diagnosis. It seems unfair to me to think of these women facing breast cancer treatment at the same time as having young children at home. Yes, younger women can become ill, but diseases like breast cancer become more common in the 40s and certainly when a woman passes 50.

And, we might add, so do heart disease and other age-related health problems in both men and women.

Women who decide to attempt pregnancy with donated eggs and who do not succeed in becoming pregnant often report a sense of failure. They say that their bodies let them down and speak of diminished self-esteem. For those who tried other ARTs before egg donation, there can be a more profound sense of failure. "Nothing seems to work. Even when there are great eggs, I still cannot become pregnant." It can be argued that these women received benefit from egg donation in that it gave them another chance at pregnancy, but harm also can be seen, since they ended the process feeling an increased sense of failure.

Another ethical consideration regarding recipients is one of justice. Should everyone have the opportunity to obtain donated eggs? If so, then we are likely to see more 60-year-old women deciding to pursue pregnancy, and we have already acknowledged some of the ways in which this may not be non-maleficent. Furthermore, recipients from certain groups—for example, lesbians, single women, low-income women and older women—may find it more difficult to access egg donation. What choices should they be allotted as far as family building is concerned? Exactly which characteristics should be used to evaluate potential egg donors? Should criteria beyond medical and reproductive health be considered? Is it appropriate to select egg donation recipients based on certain subjective criteria such as lifestyle, social status and ability to fit someone's definition of a "good" parent?

However, if certain groups are excluded as egg donor recipients, questions of justice arise. What if a particular program decides to deny access to lesbians or to single women or perhaps to people who already have children? We can easily see how access to egg donation and restricting that access can create some ethical quandaries.

Members of the extended families

The families of recipients of egg donation enjoy many benefits and so it can well be argued that egg donation is in their best interests. Grandparents get new grandchildren, cousins get cousins, aunts and uncles get nieces and nephews. The family expands and this brings happiness to many, all the more so when the new parents are known to have endured much suffering in order to become parents. On the other hand, the feelings of the donor's extended family are rarely addressed. At a recent meeting (Ellen) of mental health professionals involved in egg donation, one group member said that she "cringed" when her step-daughter said she wanted to donate eggs. Others in the group all said we could identify with her reactions. Although we help others become parents through egg donation, none of us—the potential grandparents—would want our daughters donating eggs to strangers.

The ethical question that arises for extended families is "Who am I related to?" While this is unlikely to be a problem in intrafamily donation or even friend-to-friend donation, questions do arise when a program-recruited donor provides eggs to several families. The children in those families, as well as all members of the donor's genetic family, may not know who one another are and may be cut off from contact. This may take an emotional toll and, possibly, a medical one as well, since there are instances in which genetic relatives—if they were known and in touch—might be willing to donate life-saving bone marrow or become live organ donors for one another.

Wendy Kramer, co-founder of the Donor Sibling Registry, reports that she is hearing from increasing numbers of parents of donors. These "grandparents" voice feelings about the "grandchildren" they have through egg donation. In many instances, they have no contact with these children, nor even a way to know anything about them. However, some are making connections with these children and their families and beginning to forge relationships on the DSR.

Society at large
The greatest ethical questions posed by egg donation are those that relate to our society at large. Is there benefit to society as a result of egg donation?

Surely, there are positive societal outcomes from egg donation. Egg donation brings new children into the world, some of whom may make major contributions to humankind through their work in medicine, the arts, education and more. Egg donation also enables cancer survivors and others who have suffered significant loss early in life to bear children. It offers couples in which the woman is significantly older than her husband the opportunity to share a pregnancy and raise a child together, something that has long been afforded older men and their younger wives. The world expands in many ways through the use of donated eggs, and with this expansion come many potential benefits.

What are the drawbacks? We have already addressed some of them. Payment to donors raises concerns about people and body parts becoming commodities and whole segments of the population being cut off from their genetic relatives and heritage. Prospective parents can now extend their childbearing years, bringing children into the world who may be caring for aged parents before the children themselves reach adulthood or who may be in need of care should their parents die before the children are independent.

In addition, the different approaches to egg donation worldwide have led to "fertility tourism"—people traveling from one country to another seeking eggs. Although this travel could be defended in terms of autonomy (people have an opportunity to create the families they want) and justice (people worldwide can access egg donation), ethical questions arise. Ruth Deech, author of "Reproductive tourism in Europe: infertility and human rights" (2003), explains that the rapid development of health-related technologies and the mobility and knowledge of people have led to the globalization of assisted reproductive technologies. Gametes and embryos may be passed from country to country in search of one that permits the desired treatment or allows the chosen gametes to be used. This is becoming more and more popular with egg donation, as women are becoming "fertility tourists" and paying large sums of money to travel abroad in their desperate search to find egg donors and programs that will allow them to become parents at any cost.

In his article "Unpacking the global human egg trade" (2009), author Scott Carney writes how fertility travel enables some people—such as Lavi Aron and Omer Shatzky, a gay couple in Tel Aviv—to become parents. In order to have their marriage recognized in Israel, they wed in Toronto. But the dream of having children seemed impossible. "As a gay couple, it is nearly impossible to adopt here" (2010), says Aron. "The only real option was to hire a surrogate, but oh, the cost" (2010). Friends in similar situations had found that the price of surrogacy and egg donation could easily exceed $300,000, with years of legal wrangling.

Carney goes on to say that the couple was able to become parents through Elite IVF, a Switzerland-based company which found them an egg donor in Mexico City and a US surrogate who flew to Mexico City for transfer. Two embryos were transferred—one with Aron's sperm and the other with Shatzky's, and twins—a boy and a girl—were born as American citizens. "It was like winning the lottery for us," says Aron. "Genetically, one belongs to him and one belongs to me. But they're also siblings because they come from the same egg donor. We could not have a better family than this. Everyone is connected to each other." Within weeks, Aron and Shatzky were able to arrange legal adoptions of the children and bring them back to Tel Aviv. The total cost was $120,000.

Carney writes:

Perhaps more than any other company, Elite IVF has transformed baby-making into a globalized, industrialized process. For Sher, its director, outsourcing is simply the inevitable outcome of the science that allowed procreation to move out of the bedroom and into the lab. Like the Petra Clinic and the Institut Marquès, Elite IVF offers clients cheaper access to eggs and a full suite of fertility treatments; unlike those more-localized operations, Elite operates worldwide, with offices and partner clinics in Britain, Canada, Cyprus, Israel, Mexico, Romania, and the US. Sher plans to expand soon to Turkey, taking advantage of new bans on egg donation there. (2010)

Professor Macklin (1996) looks at the issue of payment to donors and questions whether the availability of egg donation will result in wealthier couples "paying money to poorer women for the use of their bodies" (p.111). Macklin responds to this question: "All things considered, it is implausible to conclude that paying egg donors is exploitive. The facts surrounding the socioeconomic status of egg donors show that they do not come from the poorest class of society" (ibid). Still, if people are encouraged to travel from one country to another for donated eggs, there may be more opportunity for egg brokers to entice poorer women to donate eggs.

In her article "Toward a Feminist Perspective on Gamete Donation and Reception Policies" (1996), Dr. Rosemarie Tong, Thatcher Professor in Philosophy and Medical Humanities at Davidson College in North Carolina, offers another perspective on the societal impact of egg donation. Tong observes that "cultural feminists" see in egg donation (as well as in sperm donation) "possibilities for increased human connection—the kind of collaborative reproduction that, in the 1960s, was supposed to defeat the view that children are 'genetic possessions'" (p.140). Having noted this way in which egg donation contributes to a fabric of society, Tong emphasizes that feminists who hold this position insist, as we do, that donation be open and, they add, "non commercial" (p.141). She adds, "If gamete donors are interested, they should at least be kept posted on their genetic child's development, and at some point in time, perhaps when the child has reached the age of majority, at least be introduced to him or her" (p.147).

Another societal question involves the use of medical and societal resources. Although there have been some who have argued that infertility is not a disease, RESOLVE and other organizations have worked hard to educate the public and the health insurance industry so that infertility is, indeed, recognized as a serious medical condition. Nonetheless, with children worldwide needing homes, many argue that the pursuit of treatment for infertility should have its limits and that some infertile couples should be encouraged to consider adoption, not because it is their obligation but because familiarity with adoption often makes it more attractive to infertile couples.

Where does egg donation fit into the debate over the use of medical and social resources? Again, some would argue that egg donor recipients should be offering homes to children who need them rather than creating children who will be "half-adopted" anyway. Others counter and ask, "Why shouldn't a 32-year-old woman who lost her ovarian function during chemotherapy not be able to become pregnant, carry and deliver a child that is her husband's genetic offspring?" Isn't egg donation, which enables a woman to use half of her reproductive capacity, something beneficent, just and respectful of people's autonomy?

In Massachusetts, where there has been mandated coverage for infertility for many years, health insurance companies have found ways—some just and others less so—to address the question of when medical resources should be allocated for egg donation. In general, insurance will cover egg donation for any woman whose ovarian failure is premature. By contrast, insurance plans find ways of distinguishing peri-menopause and menopause from early ovarian failure and do not offer coverage in these instances. Although this leads to frustration and disappointment for some couples, it appears to adhere to medical ethics in that all those with ovarian failure that is truly premature—and, hence, a medical problem—receive the benefits of coverage.

One of the darkest sides of egg donation is that it has unleashed the possibility of "designer breeding" and thereby raises disturbing questions about eugenics. Currently, few couples have sought specific traits in selecting egg donors; there is not therefore an abnormally large proportion of, say, tall, blonde, athletic, Ivy League-bound children running around. But as egg donation becomes more widespread, these questions will become increasingly real.

It is one thing for people to select out for medical conditions, for people to decide they don't want a donor with a family history of mental retardation, depression or alcoholism. That's one of the benefits of current medical technology—to figure out what's a disease and what we can do to prevent it. But it's quite another thing for people to choose for specific enhancements and improvements.

And yet, while realizing that question must be asked for the sake of society, individuals must still make decisions. Whether one particular potential mother accepts the social stereotypes associated with education, IQ or physical appearance, and whether she pays more money to a college-educated donor than to a working-class donor, will have little impact on general patterns of social stereotyping and class division. Each individual's decision is limited in scope, and her responsibility for overall social patterns—even ones she has contributed to—is likewise limited. However, this does not mean the issues are not significant and can be ignored. Like other broad social issues—conservation, racism and so forth—each single person's actions are of little consequence, but each person's contributions are necessary to creating a solution to the problem on the large scale. Egg recipients, who object to "social engineering" on the basis of education, IQ, physical appearance and the like can be true to their values by seeking egg donors on the basis of socially neutral criteria such as overall health alone. While their contribution to the trend in general may be small, they can feel good about adhering to their own ethical and moral code.

Questions of faith

"Be fruitful and multiply"

Whether you are a Christian or a Jew, a Muslim or a member of the Buddhist or Hindu faiths, you have most likely been raised in a religion that values family and encourages its members to bring children into this world. Regardless of your faith, you probably read in your Bible or Torah or Qu'ran about the pain of infertility and the quest for children. Indeed, the pain of infertility dates back to earliest biblical times and to the recorded suffering of Sarah, Leah, Hannah, Rachel and so many others. Rachel's plaintive cry, "Give me children, or I die," has been echoed and re-echoed throughout recorded history, with people of all religions and all degrees of faith struggling with infertility.

When an individual or couple is struggling to have a child, they often find that their struggle precipitates a crisis of faith. It is not unusual to question your beliefs, your faith in God, your relationship with God and your participation in your religion. Since organized religion celebrates the arrival of children, you may find yourself avoiding your place of worship at a time when you may most need the solace of prayer. After all, who wants to enter a sanctuary, seeking comfort, only to encounter a baptism or a naming ceremony?

Similarly, you may be tempted to avoid religious holidays and celebrations. Take Easter and Passover, for example—two profoundly significant religious holidays. Each is a time when families gather together for prayer, food and a celebration of children. These holidays are made all the more poignant for their infertile participants by their central symbol: the egg. It is easy to understand why many struggling with infertility feel that they must distance themselves from religious practice, if not also from faith.

Again, volumes have been written about religion and infertility, and in his article "Religious Views Regarding Gamete Donation" (1996), Dr. Joseph Schenker narrows the focus to egg and sperm donation. Schenker examines the specific religious doctrine applicable to egg donation in the Christian (with special sections on Roman Catholicism, Eastern Orthodox, Anglican and Protestant perspectives), Jewish, Islamic, Hindu and Buddhist faiths.

We turn now to some of the central questions of faith that arise when people are considering using donated eggs.

Is God punishing me/us, and, if so, for what?

If you are considering egg donation, you may wonder whether your infertility is God's way of punishing you. But for what?

Since many of us live with regret, often around reproductive or family-building decisions, it can be easy to identify something you did wrong that generated this dreadful punishment. Some may go directly to an abortion or the decision to place a child for adoption, two of the most painful histories for those experiencing infertility. Others, who have secondary infertility, quickly conclude that they are being punished for not being good enough parents, for not fully appreciating the child or children they have, "for wanting more when we should be grateful."

For others, explanations for punishment are less clear. "Maybe it was because I focused too much on my career?" "Maybe I should have stayed with my first husband, when I was young enough to have a child, and somehow worked it out?" "Perhaps God is punishing us for intermarriage." And the list goes on.

Why is God doing this to me/us when I/we have been so good?

While some people of faith conclude that God is punishing them for some transgression, large or small, that warrants punishment, others are left baffled. They examine their behavior, past and present, and feel that they have conducted themselves in ways of which they are proud. They know that they would be good parents or are good parents deserving of another child. Unlike others who become angry at themselves for inviting this punishment, they become angry at God. In many ways, this is far more painful.

Feeling betrayed by God is extraordinarily difficult. For one thing, it shakes your faith: "How can we continue to believe in a good and just God when this happens?" For another, it estranges you from family and friends, especially from those who do not seem to lead their lives so virtuously but who are still rewarded with children. And as we said earlier, it is tempting to stay away from church, synagogue, temple or mosque when you are going through infertility. This aversion to religious services becomes all the more prominent when you feel betrayed. After all, who wants to attend a service that praises God when you are feeling let down, alone, cheated and unfairly punished?

Is this God's plan?

A question directly related to the egg donor decision is one regarding "God's plan." This is most difficult for those who believe in an all-knowing, all-giving and all-planning God. "If God has a plan for me, why does it include infertility?"

The idea of a plan may be comforting. Maybe God intends you to adopt a child? That perspective may offer some solace and some guidance in your decision making, or it can feel as if you are in a bind. What do you do if you are interested in egg donation but you believe God intends you to adopt?

For some people of faith, God's plan is something that can be flexible. You may conclude that God has a plan for you to take an alternative path to parenthood, but it is left for you to determine that plan. For example, Nina, who had just about concluded that she should adopt because that "seemed to be God's plan," reversed direction when she renewed contact with an old friend who then offered to donate eggs. From Nina's perspective, "God brought her back into my life for a reason."

At other points in this book, we have talked about "the blessing and the curse of the meant to be." Surely, it is in the area of faith that we see both sides of this perspective. It can feel like a burden to have to conform to God's plan or a blessing to believe that God has guided you in your decision and freed you from having to make decisions for yourself.

What if my religion does not support egg donation or places significant restrictions on our participation?

Religious faiths offer varying perspectives on egg donation. Although individual members of the clergy accept and support the availability of donated eggs, many faiths do attempt to limit, if not ban, the practice. According to Dr. Schenker, an expert on religious faith and professor at Hadassah University Medical Center in Jerusalem, Islam prohibits gamete donation as well as adoption. Roman Catholicism prohibits all gamete donation (1996). The Anglican church bans third-party egg or sperm donation. The Eastern Orthodox churches regard gamete donation as an adulterous act. Hinduism accepts both egg and sperm donation, as does Buddhism, as long as the child has the right to know his genetic mother or father. The Reform, Conservative and Reconstructionist movements in Judaism accept egg donation, as do several, but not all, Protestant Christian denominations. Orthodox Judaism accepts egg donation but places severe restrictions on the timing and protocol for medical diagnostic and treatment procedures. Jewish law states that "a child is related to the one who finished its formation, that is, the one who gave birth" (pp.238–250). Christian Scientists are instructed by their faith not to pursue assisted reproductive technology, including egg donation (1996).

And so we see that there will be many people of faith who find themselves in a quandary: "How do we follow the commandments of our religious tradition—to bring children into our faith—when our religion is telling us that we cannot use donated eggs?" Some conclude that they cannot turn to egg donation if their faith instructs them otherwise. However, others feel that religious doctrine can be interpreted in various ways and that the important thing is that a child will be born into a faith and raised to respect and honor it. Some are comforted in this approach by clergy or by physicians who are members of their faith and who encourage and support their actions.

Does prayer help, and, if so, how?

Prayer is comforting. Prayer offers solace. Prayer is communal. But does prayer work and, if so, how? Some people pray, seeking only one response from God. If the desired response is the birth of a child, anything else that happens feels as though one's prayers have not been answered. However, others approach prayer in a different way, feeling that the experience of praying is, in its own way, healing. In addition, they may feel that "God works in strange ways" and that this may include a different response to their prayers. Other traditions teach that prayer should ask from God only the strength to accept whatever is His will.

Some people of faith derive enormous comfort from repeating prayers that come from their tradition and that have been spoken for generations before them. Others seek to develop their own prayers, either by writing them or by combining existing prayers into something that seems to fit with their particular circumstances. In her book *Tears of Sorrow, Seeds of Hope* (1999), Rabbi Nina Cardin includes some prayers written by women and men struggling with infertility and pregnancy loss. Although some are clearly rooted in Jewish tradition, others offer words that apply to people of many faiths, regardless of their religious affiliation. Among them is this one we felt our readers might find meaningful:

> Choose from Your sacred treasury of souls and give us a child who is wise and caring, healthy and secure. May we be blessed with a pregnancy that lasts, with a birth that yields life and a child who gives us joy.
>
> May our family grow through the years and through your kindness, may we be a blessing to all who know us.
>
> May the words of our mouths and the desires of our hearts please You, our Strength and our Deliverer. (Cardin 1999, p.74)

Creating Ceremonies

In their book *Creating Ceremonies: Innovative Ways to Meet Adoption Challenges* (1999), authors Cheryl Lieberman and Rhea Bufferd talk about the value of creating ceremonies for adoptive families, a concept that has been borrowed by many who have built their families through other alternative means, including egg donation. Included in the ceremonies Lieberman and Bufferd refer to are ceremonies of celebration. Although Lieberman and Bufferd's ceremonies are not religious in nature, the idea of creating rituals and ceremonies is one familiar and comforting to people of faith.

If you bring a child into your family through donated eggs, you will surely want to participate in your faith's rituals and ceremonies around birth and infancy. Baptisms, Bris and Naming Ceremonies are all sacred events that confirm that a child is authentically a member of your family and your faith. In addition to celebrating these long-awaited occasions, you may want to create some of your own ceremonies. For example, adoptive families sometimes bring home some soil from the place they adopted their child and mix that soil with the soil in their yard, planting in it a tree or flowers. You may want to find some way to similarly honor and celebrate your egg donor and your experience with her.

For many couples, the crisis of faith that arises during their infertility experience and their egg donor journey actually serves to strengthen their religious connections. Just as infertility will challenge, but usually not destroy, strong relationships, so also can it shake, but not destroy, religious faith. Some find that they are comforted, fortified and renewed by prayer. Others receive enormous support and guidance from clergy or from other members of their faith. And many draw strength from knowing that the birth of a child will bring delight to their families, who will join them in welcoming that child into their family.

– 10 –

The Globalization of Egg Donation

The first baby conceived through donated eggs was born in Australia in 1983. Within a short time, there were clinics worldwide offering some form of egg donation. Local laws, customs and beliefs led to widely varying practices from one country to another. Because egg donation remains a rapidly changing field and one with widely divergent laws and practices from one county to another, a summary of egg donation worldwide is beyond the scope of this book. However, we do feel that it is important to address one increasingly common phenomenon: travel for egg donation.

"Fertility tourism" is the somewhat offputting term used in reference to people who travel for egg donation. We call it offputting because "tourism" has been defined as "the commercial organization and operation of vacations and visits to places of interest" (New Oxford American Dictionary). We challenge anyone who sees someone seeking a resolution of infertility as going on vacation. Yes, people are traveling for egg donation and a lucky few get to enjoy a pleasant visit in a place that interests them, but having a vacation is never the primary reason for their journey.

Why, then, do people travel for egg donation? The following are the most common reasons people travel for egg donation:

- cost

- legal restrictions in the recipient's home country

- ethical considerations

- the family story

- chance of success.

Cost

At the time of writing, someone seeking egg donation in the US faces costs upwards of $30,000 for one cycle. Donor agencies vary in their fees, as do medical programs, lawyers and psychologists. Some recipients are fortunate enough to have coverage for some of the costs through their health insurance.

There are many people who cannot afford egg donation in the US. Prompted by lower costs in South Africa, the Czech Republic, Spain, India, Barbados and elsewhere, people are traveling for egg donation. To give you some sense of the difference in costs, at the time of writing, the total cost for a US couple to travel to South Africa for egg donation, staying ten days, is about $17,000, The cost to travel to the Czech Republic averages $6500 for treatment plus another $2000 for airfare, hotel and food. Fees vary from program to program within these countries and travel costs also vary, but it's easy to see, from these numbers, that traveling for egg donation saves a good deal of money.

Olivia Montuschi, co-founder (with her husband, Walter) of the Donor Conception Network in the United Kingdom observes that, in the UK also, people often travel abroad because of lower costs and greater availability of donors. However, one way that costs are kept down in the UK is through egg sharing, a practice by which women going through IVF agree to share their eggs with another woman for a combination of financial and altruistic reasons. Usually, the donor will have a free or heavily subsidized cycle in return for egg sharing. The women having IVF have to be under 35 and having treatment for a condition not related to egg quality. Clinics all have strict protocols about how the egg sharing works. In most cases, if a woman produces fewer than six eggs, they are not shared but stay with the donor. If she produces an uneven number, then the donor gets the extra one. All women contemplating egg sharing have to be counseled about the implications of doing so. This is taken very seriously as, in the UK, donors become identifiable to offspring from age 18. Currently, egg sharing accounts for around 60 percent of the donated eggs in the UK.

Legal restrictions

Egg donation is banned in some countries and in others there are limitations on who can participate in egg donation, with exclusions to single women and lesbian couples. Other countries ban payment to donors, limiting the number of available donors, and some countries ban anonymity. Restrictions in one's home country are prompting increasing numbers of intended parents to travel abroad for egg donation.

Israeli women commonly travel abroad for egg donation. There are almost no donors in Israel as only women who have undergone fertility treatment can donate. Women seeking egg donation undergo an induction process in Israel in order to prepare their uterus to receive eggs. There are Israeli physicians who are in close contact with physicians abroad and travel with their patients, most often to the Czech Republic or to Cyprus, Romania or Russia. Women pay for the treatment themselves but receive some reimbursement by the Israeli government and permission to bring any remaining embryos back to Israel for transfer in a subsequent cycle. (Ironically, there are many young Israeli women who donate eggs but do so abroad, usually to earn money when they are traveling.)

Ethical considerations

Ethical considerations are another reason that some intended parents travel for egg donation. Some people living in the US are troubled by the high fees that are paid to donors and/or by the widespread practice of anonymity. They are concerned also that medical programs in the US may be giving donors too much medication in an effort to push their ovaries to produce lots of eggs. Some recipients travel because they worry about the medical care their donor is receiving and feel that she is less likely to face hyperstimulation abroad. One woman, who traveled from the US to the Czech Republic reported talking with her physicians both at home and in Prague about how much medication they give donors.

One US-based program that facilitates egg donation in South Africa, Barbados and India is Global Egg Donors. Founder and director Robin Newman says that it is important to her not to over-pay her donors nor to work with clinics that overstimulate them. Donors for Global Egg Donors receive payment of $750, a modest amount considering how much time and effort is devoted to this endeavor. Newman says that she feels confident that this sum removes payment as a motivation for egg donation.

Another ethical reason to travel for egg donation involves the number of times someone donates. Although we are told in the US that payment is for time and effort, not eggs, women typically receive higher payments if they are proven donors, meaning they have successfully donated before. As a result, there is financial incentive to donate multiple times, something that does not exist in many programs outside the US.

Robin Newman raises another ethical concern about many of the programs in the US. She notes that, in most instances, women do not have a say in choosing the family they are donating to. Programs will ask a woman to say whether she is willing to donate to same-sex couples or to singles, but, beyond weighing in on these broad categories, she does not get to make more specific choices such as donating only to a childless couple or to one in which the woman will carry the baby. By contrast, participants in Global Egg Donors are required to write a letter to a prospective donor introducing themselves and asking her if she is willing to donate to them. This exchange helps confirm that this is truly a gift from one family to another and not a sale or business transaction.

The family story

As we have stressed throughout this book, parents through egg donation create a story for their child. In building that story, they want to make decisions that they will feel good about in the future. Choosing to travel for egg donation addresses several aspects of the family story. In addition to removing/reducing concerns about payment to the donor and of multiple donations, intended parents have the opportunity to travel to a place that is meaningful to them. In some instances, this place may represent their heritage and, in others, may simply add to the richness of their journey. Nearly everyone who goes through egg donation refers to their process as a journey and, by traveling to a foreign land, many get to experience a meaningful sojourn in a distant land. This has been felt by some of have traveled to India, in particular.

I (Ellen) have a client who has Eastern European heritage and who conceived her beloved child in Prague. As someone whose identity is very much connected to her cultural heritage and who is married to man who shares that heritage, the opportunity to go to Prague made all the difference in enabling her to fully embrace egg donation. Spending a week or so there transformed an experience that began as one of loss into one that brought unexpected rewards. She returned home pregnant and with a host of memories to one day share with her child.

Another of my clients (Ellen) is of Indian heritage, with much of her large extended family living in India. There are Indian donors in the US, but she prefers to travel to India for several reasons. In addition to the cost being significantly lower, this intended mom feels more comfortable with the story she will have for her child. Aware that a child conceived through egg donation (like all children) will one day be sorting out his identity, my client likes the fact that she will be able to speak of his Indian heritage with authenticity and also, a sense of pride about where he came from. In addition, she and her husband will be able to stay with her grandmother when they go to India, something they rarely get to do. The intended mom observes that this visit will be one of the unexpected bonuses of egg donation.

Chance of success

Finally, there is the matter of whether it will work. For some recipients, the decision to travel for egg donation is based on their understanding of their chances for success. For example, one British woman tells of her decision to go to Spain for egg donation nine years ago. At that time she had several reasons for traveling, most of which involved chances for success. She found that the donors in Spain were younger than in the UK and she was advised that the clinic she was considering in Madrid was more up-to-date medically than the one available to her in the UK. The following is an excerpt from an essay by a DC Network member, written after giving birth to her daughter:

> Lloyd and I had always wished that the donors in the UK and Spain weren't anonymous. We were unsure what to do. On one hand the clinic was just about to match us, Lloyd's sperm was already in Spain and all the papers were signed. On the other hand it was very important to us that any child born from a donor egg should have the right to know about their heritage and have the chance to meet their donor if they wished.
>
> If I cancelled the Spanish treatment I'd have to get on to a UK list which were already around 2–4 years long before the law change announcement. The feeling was that the lists would get even longer as it was assumed that some women may now not want to donate or egg share if they thought any children from a donation could contact them! The media was full of shock horror headlines about donor shortages and extensive waiting lists! It now seemed that a probable three-year wait had suddenly become a four- or five-year wait. Even if I could get myself on to a UK list and successfully advertise for a donor, the wait would be at least another two years as the new law wasn't due to come into force for another year.
>
> Our clinic in Spain had told us we'd only have to wait another three weeks to start down regulating…it was all about to happen after so

many years and so many disappointments. Our chance of becoming parents was tantalizingly close.

We considered everything very carefully: the removal of anonymity in the UK would lead to a situation in the future where children born from UK egg donors would be in a very different situation to children of the same age born from anonymous donors abroad… was this acceptable?

We also discussed the issues surrounding donor compensation. It's illegal to pay donors for their eggs in Spain but the clinics "compensate" egg donors by around 800 Euros—roughly £500 [$800]. The majority of the donors are students and Lloyd and I felt that £500 was a reasonable amount of compensation to receive for egg donation, especially as the cost of living in Madrid is very high. We did not feel that £500 was an amount that would lead to the exploitation of donors as it might do in countries where the cost of living is much lower. But of course we have no way of knowing the individual circumstances of the donors.

Concerns about traveling for egg donation

We turn now to reasons why individuals and couples would choose not to travel for egg donation.

Donor evaluation

If you decide to travel for egg donation, you will want some reassurance that the donors available to you in your host country are women who have been thoroughly evaluated, both medically and psychologically. Medical tests should help ensure that donors are in overall good health and free from genetic conditions that could be transmitted to a child. Psychological testing attempts to rule out women who have serious mental illness as well as those whose current situations suggest it is unwise to donate at this time.

Ellie Goldman, LICSW, who spoke with many prospective donors while she was working for a busy US agency, recalls being struck by how few of the women actually ended up going through with the process. Her estimate is that only 10–15 percent of those who expressed initial interest in donating actually entered the process and moved on to medical and psychological screening (where some were "screened out" for medical or psychological issues or both). Some of those who dropped out after expressing interest or were screened out early on included women who had BMIs (body mass index) outside of the "normal" range, women who had a lot going on in their lives, making this a difficult time for them to commit to egg donation, women who took several weeks to get back to the program after initial contact, women who said they wanted to donate because they have "great genes" and those who planned to keep donation a secret from close family. Other red flags include women who don't seem prepared for their interviews and who lack a basic understanding of the process and those who have recently experienced a major loss including the break-up of a relationship, the death of a loved one, an abortion or miscarriage. Goldman adds that many women screen themselves out early on because they don't understand how time-consuming and invasive the medical process is and those who find themselves having unanticipated thoughts and feelings about having donor offspring "out in the world."

Lack of counseling

There are programs that provide excellent medical care but do so in the absence of any required counseling for donors or recipients. Although many people don't like being told that counseling is required, most find it helpful. Often donors and recipients will comment that the counselor brought up things they had never thought of. Undergoing medical treatment at a program that doesn't require counseling poses a twofold risk: you may be receiving eggs from a young woman who hasn't fully explored her feelings about gamete donation and you yourselves may think you have covered everything but later look back and wonder why you didn't more fully explore some aspect of this decision.

Limited information

In the US, even those who choose anonymous egg donation know a great deal about their donors. They generally have photographs of her and her family. There are extensive questionnaires, both medical and social, and recipients often have the opportunity to ask her additional questions through the agency. Programs in Spain and the Czech Republic, for example, offer little information. In fact, there are clinics that reportedly refuse to give any information about their donors beyond their age and blood type.

Throughout this book we have tried to respectfully raise our concerns about anonymity. Having donors about whom almost nothing is known raises these concerns exponentially.

Cultural identity

Most people have feelings about where they came from. In the melting pot of the US, we have people who are proudly Italian or Greek, Polish or Danish. People regard their cultural identity as an important piece of who they are. This goes for "Italians" who have never been to Italy and "French Canadians" who have never been north of New York City.

What does it mean to be disconnected from one's cultural identity? Some people travel for egg donation because they seek a specific culture, such as a person who has Eastern European heritage and intentionally travels to Prague for a donor. However, some who travel do not have any connection to the culture of the donor and, in some instances, they do not even know what it is. Spanish clinics, for example, are reportedly recruiting donors from Eastern Europe.

I (Ellen) interviewed one father through egg donation who joined his own family through adoption who said:

> As an adoptee with a birth father who was a West Indian, I can vouch for the importance of knowing where my land is, of the uncanny sense of familiarity, home and peace that for me is unique to the West Indies.

Quality of medical care

By all reports, the medical care for egg donation is excellent in many clinics throughout the world. Fear of not getting good medical care in another country is not a reason to stay at home. However, most people feel more confident in their ability to assess the medical care in their home country because there are no language or cultural barriers to overcome. Traveling for egg donation often means doing some advanced research on the laboratory standards and screening of donors at a clinic in another country.

Laws vary from country to country, but many clinics follow the same guidelines for testing that are utilized in the United States. European clinics typically comply with the rigorous European Union guidelines for STD testing as well as genetic illnesses and psychological factors, although the details of what may be ruled out are not disclosed as in the United States.

For a variety of reasons, including their strict parameters used for testing, the Czech Republic has become one of the most popular destinations for third-party reproduction.

The Czech Republic has a strong Ministry of Health that oversees all aspects of STD testing prior to treatment, procedures related to storage of eggs, sperms and embryos, and any transport laws regulating the handling of tissues, shipping of sperm and embryos. Since the development of European Union laws in 2010, the Czech Republic clinics are also subject to the European tissue directive which impacts IVF methods and donation of reproductive cells.

Donor selection

In the US, recipients choose their donors and have the option to choose donors who are willing to meet them. Even those who choose anonymous donors do so based on extensive information provided by the donor and, often, the agency. This is not always the case abroad, where the clinic doctors may do the matching. Having seen how seriously intended parents in the US take donor selection and how much pleasure they get from finding someone who feels right, we have concerns about what it means to have someone else—and in this instance, a virtual stranger—make lasting decisions about one's family. Physicians are likely to select donors based on physical resemblance and likely fertility, and while both are important criteria for almost all recipients, they represent only a portion of what people focus on. We have so often found that when intended parents are looking at donors, what seems to matter most is character and personality. Recipients are so often drawn to someone because of something she wrote in her profile, by some altruistic or family-centered activity she is involved in or by her smile or her upbeat nature. Having a physician make a match means that all these deeply personal reactions to someone's personality and character are lost in the process.

Another consideration is the donor's ethnicity and how her appearance may reflect that ethnicity. While some recipients travel specifically to have a donor of a certain ethnicity, those traveling for cost or other reasons may find that the donors have "a look" that seems "foreign" to them. And what if parents are surprised to find that their child has some unexpected features? Of course this could happen in any family but, with donor conception, it can be unsettling.

How will children feel knowing that half their genetic heritage is abroad? While this may offer some comfort to some, who are less likely to be concerned that they will be dating half siblings or first cousins, we wonder how this piece of the puzzle may affect identity? Perhaps some donor offspring will feel special knowing their donor and her family are in the Czech Republic or Spain, but might others feel a sense of disconnection or displacement. In addition, those who seek some contact with donor siblings are likely to find this more difficult, if not impossible. If the doctor selects the donor and provides little information, offspring cannot turn to the Donor Sibling Registry or follow other paths to contacting siblings. Even those who can make contact may be thwarted from in-person visits by long-distance geography.

Cultural differences

With increasing numbers of people traveling across borders and sometimes across continents for egg donation, awareness of and sensitivity to cultural differences is all the more important. We are aware that we are writing from a cultural perspective that strives to avoid/reduce secrecy and which values openness and honesty within families. However, we are aware that in some cultures, there is no harm seen in having a secret in a family. These cultures include Spain, France, Italy, Romania, Portugal, Ireland, Israel, Japan, South Korea, Turkey and most South American and African countries. In conversations with egg donation recipients worldwide, we always try to "get" the cultural context before offering information or advice that is deeply rooted in our own culture.

Donor Sibling Registry co-founder, Wendy Kramer, together with her son, Ryan, was pleased to be invited to Japan. The Kramers were intrigued to see that even in the Japanese culture, where blood ties are considered of paramount importance in families, there is increased awareness of the value of openness and honesty in donor conception.

Making plans to travel for egg donation

The websites www.novasans.com or www.globalivf.com offer information about programs in the following countries: Argentina, Australia, Barbados, Brazil, Canada, Cyprus, France, Georgia, Greece, Hungary, India, Indonesia, Japan, Jordan, Kuwait, Lebanon, Malaysia, Mexico, New Zealand, Philippines, Poland, Russia, Saudi Arabia, Singapore, South Africa, South Korea, Spain, Taiwan, Thailand, Turkey, Ukraine and the United Arab Emirates.

If you are thinking about traveling to another country for egg donation, it is important that you learn something about how that culture understands and approaches the process.

– 11 –

Egg Donation,
Ever Changing

Change. One of the biggest challenges, and perhaps the greatest pleasure, in writing this book has been to participate in—and to try to keep pace with—change. News about developments in reproductive medicine and family building comes almost on a daily basis. No sooner did we write that "egg freezing is not available" in the first edition of this book than the news came out that doctors were achieving successful pregnancies with frozen eggs. And it was around the time that we were writing about "special circumstances" that gay marriage became legal in Massachusetts. As we go to press again, we have little doubt that readers will read this book a year or two or three from now and note that much of what we say is dated.

Much changes. Some things remain the same. As we look to the future, we hope for certain changes—donor registries, guaranteed access to genetic family information for recipients, widespread acceptance of donors' rights to know the outcome of their donations. Overall, we hope that secrecy around egg donation will vanish and that the shame it generated will be replaced by pride, satisfaction and gratitude.

Egg freezing

Egg freezing was first made available to young women undergoing chemotherapy or facing other medical problems that could compromise their ovarian function in the future. However, the process is also sought by women such as Jennifer Anderson, 40, interviewed on National Public Radio on October 19, 2012, who fear that their biological clock will run out before they find a life partner and are in a position to have children "the traditional way." Anderson speaks of the anxiety she felt dating prior to freezing eggs and of the relief she felt once she had frozen eggs.

In the fall of 2012 the ASRM announced that egg freezing is no longer considered experimental. This news was welcomed by many, especially single women concerned about their biological time clocks. However, the news is more complicated than it first appears. What ASRM is saying is that fertilization and pregnancy rates are encouraging when eggs are frozen via vitrification. Vitrification freezes the egg more quickly so ice crystals, which would otherwise destroy the cell's structure, do not have time to form.

There remain many unanswered questions with regard to who benefits from egg freezing. Data on pregnancy and live births from egg freezing in cancer patients are very limited. Similarly, there are no data on the efficacy of egg freezing for women over the age of 35, and data on the safety, cost-effectiveness and emotional risks for elective egg freezing to defer childbearing are insufficient as well. Although the success of egg freezing has improved dramatically and preliminary data are encouraging, it is still not a viable option for all women. Overall, egg freezing is still limited to just a few clinics, and success rates typically only include young, highly selected populations. Additionally, it is still too early to conclude anything about the long-term risks with regard to the incidence of anomalies and developmental abnormalities of children born from frozen eggs.

How successful egg freezing will be remains uncertain. No one can predict how well eggs will thaw and what the chances of a healthy pregnancy will be. However, having the technology available is attractive to young women like Ms. Anderson. In some instances, their parents are offering to pay for the procedure, generally costing between $8000 and $10,000, to ensure they will become grandparents. Rachel Lehmann-Haupt, author of *In Her Own Sweet Time: Unexpected Adventures in Finding Love,*

Commitment, and Motherhood (2009), describes this as "the postmodern, adult birds-and-the-bees talk" in an interview on Talk To the Nation. She warns, "There is a very fine line between concern and pressure." Plus, age is an important factor in the success of frozen eggs. Many women consider this option only as a last resort and don't really start looking into it seriously until their late 30s or early 40s when the viability of their eggs has significantly decreased. In any case, egg freezing will most likely continue to expand as technologies improve.

Frozen egg banks

The ability to successfully freeze eggs has also brought frozen egg banks, a new source of donated eggs. Egg banks invite intended parents to choose them over "traditional" egg donation, highlighting the lower cost, less stressful process, and in some instances, higher success rates. Each of these factors is compelling to intended parents, many of whom have struggled for years and whose financial and emotional resources are depleted. We are sensitive to each of these factors and can understand why recipients are and will be drawn to egg banks. However, what the banks omit in their ads is the downside of frozen banks: the human and collaborative connection between donors and recipients is diminished. At this point in time, donors and recipients are not able to meet, nor are they exchanging letters or communicating in some way through the donor agency.

Appearing on National Public Radio (NPR), Marcy Darnovsky, of the Center for Genetics and Society, suggested that egg banks could lead to the exploitation of poor, younger women. Darnovsky said, "It's pretty evident that there is usually a difference in socioeconomic status between women who are being asked to sell their eggs or rent their wombs and the women using it." NPR also turned to noted bioethicist Adrienne Asch of Yeshiva University who said egg freezing is "an example of using technology to solve social problems."

Advancing reproductive technologies

With advancing reproductive technologies, some believe that egg donation will no longer be necessary in the near future. Women will be able to become pregnant using other methods, allowing them to maintain genetic ties with their children regardless of their ovarian function.

While not widely available and still very experimental, many believe cytoplasmic or mitochondrial transfer allows another option for those considering egg donation. This is a form of assisted reproductive technology where the cytoplasm from a donor egg is injected into an egg with compromised mitochondria. The resulting egg is then fertilized with sperm and transferred to the uterus. This method was created to aid women who experience infertility due to damaged or deficient mitochondria which normally occurs as eggs age. Instead of using donor eggs, these women would be able to have a tiny bit of donor DNA injected into their own eggs. Only a few children have been born via this procedure in the last ten years. These children still have a small amount (probably 1%) of their DNA come from the donor. There are no data as to the health of children as they get older, especially with regard to serious genetic defects such as diabetes, ALS and pervasive developmental disorders. Additionally, this type of DNA transfer brings up a number of legal, ethical and moral questions related to further manipulating embryos and creating so-called genetic hybrids. Research on cytoplasmic or mitochondrial transfers has been stymied in the United States due to federal regulations, so most procedures are done abroad.

Ovarian tissue transplants have also received a lot of attention as an alternative to egg donation. Some clinics are attempting this, including in the United States, and some doctors claim that women could remain fertile indefinitely after successful ovarian transplants. Ovarian transplant is a technique to remove a piece of the ovary, store it for years and then with delicate surgery, replace it putting a woman's menopause "on ice," so to speak.

Researchers report that more than 20 babies have now been born worldwide to patients who have had their own ovarian tissue removed before treatment that would have left them infertile, and replaced it afterwards, or, in another case, where one twin donated ovarian tissue to the other. Moreover, most of these children have been conceived naturally after the transplant without the need for IVF, fertility drugs or any other interventions. To date, all the women who have undergone ovarian transplants have had cancer, but many think it is now time to expand this technique to others.

Dr. Sherman Silber, an American reproductive endocrinologist practicing in St. Louis, Missouri, states that women wanting to stave off menopause "could have grafts removed as a young women and then have the first replaced as you approach menopausal age. You can then put a slice back every decade" (Adams 2012). It is still unclear how long ovarian transplants remain viable for women to become pregnant on their own; some say just few months and others say indefinitely. Although this is an exciting new development in reproductive medicine, we need a lot more data to understand the long-term outcomes. Also, it is not known about possible effects on cancer, heart disease, osteoporosis and menopause. The first ovarian transplant was done in 2003, and we are still many years away from knowing if this is a realistic option.

The rights of donor offspring

The rights of children to have access to their genetic history has been a concern for many years. First stemming from the adoption community, the importance of genetic links is now being seen among children of sperm donors who are searching for their donor dads. Because adoption laws allowing for information about biological parents do not apply to donated gametes, legal cases have emerged arguing that all children have the right to know their parents and that children of sperm donors should not be discriminated against.

Because sperm donation has been around for decades and many more children have been born via sperm donation, these children have been leading the way in this area. However, issues are similar among children conceived by egg donor, especially as they get older and their numbers grow, and it is just a matter of time before these children have the same needs and desires with regard to their own genetic information.

On May 19, 2011, the Supreme Court of British Columbia issued a landmark ruling supporting the rights of donor offspring. This ruling came in response to a law suit brought by Olivia Pratten, conceived in 1981 though donor sperm. Ms. Pratten had spent years of fruitless efforts trying to identify her sperm donor and, when all else failed, sued the provincial government, arguing that the law discriminated against children of egg and sperm donation because they don't have the same ability as adopted children to learn about their genetic roots.

The May ruling granted a permanent injunction against the destruction of donor records in BC and gave that government 15 months to amend laws to address the rights of donor offspring. Sadly the ruling was overturned in November 2012 on appeal, but Ms. Pratten may take the case to the country's top court, according to Canadian media reports.

On July 22, 2011, the State of Washington passed legislation that significantly reduces anonymity in egg and sperm donation. Unless egg and sperm donors exercise their right to withhold their identify, donor offspring now have access to their donor's identity. This law, while limited, is an important step forward and paves the way for more legislation ensuring the rights of donor-conceived people in the US and Canadian provinces.

Because donors can easily opt out, it is unclear whether this law will have much practical impact. Still, assisted reproduction attorney Mark Demaray says it's a step. "At least it requires the clinics to have a conversation with any donor," he says. "So they need to think about what that means 18 years from now. And I think that's a good discussion to have for both recipient families and for donors" (Ludden 2011).

While, for some, interest is sparked by curiosity and a need to understand their life narrative, it also might be a matter of life or death. In my (Evelina) own family, we recently faced an unexpected, early and potentially life-threatening cancer diagnosis, even though we had absolutely no family history of cancer before this. We also found that this rare cancer occurrence most likely had genetic links almost certainly passed on to our children. Fortunately, with extensive genetic testing and regular screenings starting as teenagers, we can detect it early, preventing our children from getting a similar cancer. Had we been gamete donors, this would have been critical information for any donor children to have in order to protect their health. Without a registry, there would be no way for us to pass along this life-saving information.

Dr. Jennifer Schneider experienced a similar situation when her previously young and healthy daughter was diagnosed with a fatal colon cancer just four years after her egg donation (Schneider 2008). After her daughter's death, it was impossible for Dr. Schneider to get information about her daughter's donation and any biological children. The conflict often lies with the financial interest of the program versus the welfare of the donor and the children that are born. As a result, Dr. Schneider advocates for improved recommendations for further egg donor follow-up, research and actions by professional associations and regulatory agencies to ensure information sharing.

Not surprisingly, many donor-conceived families are concerned about the impact introducing this new information will have on their children and their own family dynamics. Susan Golombok, professor at the Centre for Family Research at the University of Cambridge, states that whatever the shape of modern families, the quality of the relationships is more important than the structure (Golombok *et al.* 2011). Her longitudinal studies have repeatedly shown that children who lack a genetic relationship with a parent—through egg donation, sperm donation and/or surrogacy—do very well. A parent is someone who has a relationship with a child, who brings up a child, not someone who donates DNA. Golombok has found that having a social relationship with multiple parents is not detrimental to children. Often parents think that it will be more problematic for children than it turns out to be. The more research that is done in this area, the more it supports the conclusion that "unusual" family structures often produce better relationships because these are the parents who really want to have children—that's very important.

The internet, social media, the arts and egg donation

With the advent the internet and social media, they way we gather and share information has changed dramatically. Suddenly, the world seems much smaller as we are able to find things out about people that were never before possible, often based on just a few vague clues. This can both work toward our advantage and our detriment according to the situation.

In terms of egg donation, we can search through countless egg donor programs and solicit feedback about individuals' experiences almost instantaneously. We have access to literally hundreds, if not thousands, of potential donor profiles. The egg donation process is increasingly familiar and transparent as people share intimate details about how they coped physically and mentally through Facebook, Twitter and personal blogs, as if we were right there with them every step of the way. We form virtual support groups, providing encouragement to others as they navigate the unknown. As we have seen above, the internet and social media have allowed grassroots donor registries and even individuals on their own to bridge genetic gaps often through a quick Google search. A popular infertility blogger pointed out how strange it was that so many people, many of whom she would never meet, knew all the details of her struggles with infertility and her choice to build her family through egg donation long before her future children would even be born, not to mention would even think about how they were conceived. Whether we like it or not, the internet and social media help shape our family stories.

Egg donation and other alternative paths to parenthood have also found their way into film, theater and television. For example, playwright Claire Burns draws upon her own experiences as an egg donor in her play *Hatched*, which premiered in Toronto on November 2, 2012. Burns describes the play as being "about the need to belong."

And so we come to the end of this book, knowing that our readers will be traveling down different paths to parenthood and to life after infertility. Some of our readers will choose adoption or perhaps living without children or may remain a one-child family. We hope that this book has helped you feel clearer and more secure in those decisions.

We know, also, that many of our readers will choose egg donation, and, for you, we are grateful to be able to offer some advice from one who truly knows and understands egg donation. Daniel at age 16 several years ago was asked to write about what it meant to be conceived through donated eggs. He generously shares his thoughts with you.

> There is no such thing as a perfect child, so no matter what you do, they will screw up a few times. What you should do early is to have the child develop self-esteem. That was one of the most important things I have ever been taught to be. To feel good about yourself means that you will have a brighter look on life. Self-esteem will become important when you feel nervous about people finding out how you were born. But that is not in most times true. DE in my life has really not been a big deal. I am going to live the same and die the same no matter what the heck I was born with. I just want all mothers to know that their child is no different. When I told one of my friends that I was one of the first 11 children ever conceived through DE, he said, "Um... Huh?" So tell your child that he doesn't have to worry about fitting in.
>
> Start early and start little by little telling the kids how they were conceived. If you disagree, I might be wrong because I can only say what worked for me. I think it would be worth a try though. I think one of the best ways to explain it is to put it in words they can easily understand and then, as they mature, tell them more finite details.

Donor egg is just the way I got here, but now I'm just me. I hope moms and dads who used donor eggs will feel good about the way they have their kids and good about their kids.

Thank you, Daniel, you have said it all.

RESOURCES

There are so many resources related to egg donation and the list is growing. There are books for adults, lots for children, websites, support groups and videos. We have compiled a brief sampling of some of the resources available to you.

Books and articles for adults

Alpern, K. (ed) (1992) *The Ethics of Reproduction*. New York, NY: Oxford University Press.

Bernstein, A.C. (1994) *Flight of the Stork: What Children Think (And When) about Sex and Family Building*. Indianapolis, IN: Perspective Press/St. Paul, MN: Koryo Company.

Blyth, E. and Landau, R. (2004) *Third Party Conception Across Cultures: Social, Legal and Ethical Perspectives*. London: Jessica Kingsley Publishers.

Blyth, E., Kramer, W. and Schneider, J. (2012)"Perspectives, experiences and choices of parents of children conceived following oocyte donation." *Reproductive BioMedicine Online 26*, 2, 179–188.

Cohen, C.B. (1996) *New Ways of Making Babies: The Case of Egg Donation*. Bloomington, IN: Indiana University Press.

Crockin, S.L. and Jones, H.W., Jr. (2010) *Legal Conceptions: The Evolving Law and Policy of Assisted Reproductive Technologies*. Baltimore, MD: The Johns Hopkins University Press.

Daniels, K. (2004) *Building a Family with the Assistance of Donor Insemination*. Auckland, New Zealand: Dunmore Publishing.

Daniels, K. (2007) "Donor Gametes: Anonymous or identified." *Best Practice and Research Clinical Obstetrics and Gynaecology 21*, 1, 113–28.

Ehrensaft, D. (2005) *Mommies, Daddies, Donors, Surrogates: Answering Tough Questions and Building Strong Families*. New York, NY: Guilford Press.

Glazer, E.S. (1998) *Experiencing Infertility: Stories to Inform and Inspire*. San Francisco, CA: Jossey Bass.

Kirkman, M. (2004) "Genetic connection and relationships in narratives of donor assisted conception." *Australian Journal of Emerging Technologies and Society 2*, 2, 1–20.

Kirkman, M. (2008) "Being a 'real' mum: motherhood through donated eggs and embryos." *Women's Studies International Form 31*, 4, 241–48.

Kramer, W. (2011) "Gamete donation: medical and genetic implications." *Infertiliy Updates 3*, 3, 20–1.

Lorbach, C. (2009) *Experiences of Donor Conception: Parents, Offspring and Donors through the Years*. London: Jessica Kingsley Publishers.

McWhinnie, A. (2006) *Who Am I? Experiences of Donor Conception*. Leamington Spa: Idreos Education Trust.

Morrisette, M. (2008) *Choosing Single Motherhood: The Thinking Woman's Guide*. New York, NY: Mariner Books.

Sauer, M.V. (1998) *Principles of Oocyte and Embryo Donation*. New York, NY: Springer.

Shidlo, R. (2012) "In Search of Donor Relations and Identity: The Missing Voices of Israel's Children" *Medicine and Law Journal, 31*, 641-659.

Uroz, V. and Guerra, L. (2009) "Donation of Eggs in Assisted Reproduction and Informed Consent." *Medicine and Law 28*, 565–75.

Wilson-Miller, W. and Napoletano, E. (2012) *The Insider's Guide to Egg Donation: A Compassionate and Comprehensive Guide for All Parents-to-Be*. New York, NY: Demos Health.

Books for children

Andrie, N.L. (2012) *Jhwee and Jhwah*. CreateSpace Independent Publishing Platform.

Bowder, T. (2005) *How You Came to Us*. Trafford Publishing.

Cahill, K. (2001) *I love You This Much*. Trafford Publishing.

Carswell, N. (2012) *A Very Special Lady: A Story about IVF, an Egg Donor and a Little Girl*. CreateSpace Independent Publishing Platform.

Carter, K. (2008) *What Matters Most: A Children's Book of Families*. BookSurge Publishing.

Celcer, I. and Gatto, H. (2007) *Hope and Will Have a Baby: The Gift of Egg Donation*. Jackson Heights, NY: Graphite Press.

Daniels, K. (2005) *The Baby About to Be Born: A Story of Spirit for Adoptive and ART Families*. Self-published.

Ellen, N. (2009) *The Egg Lady*. Jupiter, FL: Bittersweet Books.

Garcia, D.O. (2010) *As Many Children as the Stars*. Mustang, OK: Tate Publishing.

Gordon, E. (2011) *Mommy, Did I Grow in Your Tummy? Where Many Babies Come From*. Santa Monica, CA: EM Greenberg Press.

Grimes, J. (2004) *Before You Were Born: Our Wish for a Baby*. Webster, IA: X, Y, and Me Books.

Jover, C.M. and Martinez, R. (2005) *A Tiny Bitsy Gift of Life: An Egg Donor Story*. Self-published.

Kluger-Bell, K. (2012) *The Pea that Was Me: An Egg Donation Story*. CreateSpace Independent Publishing Platform.

Nadel, C. (2007) *Mommy, Was Your Tummy Big?* Arlington, VA: Mookind Press.

Noble, K. and Gibson, S. (2009) *One More Giraffe*. Self-published.

Prezani, S. (2012) *Sacha, The Little Bright Shooting Star: The Story of Surrogacy*. Sofia Prezani.

Shackleton, S. and Coulson, G. (2010) *Tabitha and Timothy Grow a Flower*. CreateSpace Independent Publishing Platform.

Silverberg, C. (2013) *What Makes a Baby: A Book for Kids Conceived All Kinds of Ways*. New York: Triangle Square.

Smith, C., Bainbridge, S. and Bainbridge, B. (2011) *The Hen that Couldn't Lay an Egg*. Frederick, MD: PublishAmerica.

Stamm, L. (2010) *Phoebe's Family: A Story about Egg Donation*. Jackson Heights, NY: Graphite Press.

Summer, M. (2010) *Mom and Dad and the Journey They Had*. CreateSpace Independent Publishing Platform.

Silverberg, C. and Smith, F. (2013) *What Makes a Baby: A Book for Kids Conceived All Kinds of Ways*. Triangle Square Publishing.

Throen, P. and Rinaldi, T. (2012) *Woher manche Babys Kommen: Ein Erklärungs- und Aufklärungsbuch für Kinder, die mit medizinischer Unterstützung gezeugt wurden* (in German). Germany: FamART Verlag.

Tisseron, S. and Guillerey, A. (2008) *Le Mystère des grains à bébé* (in French). France: Jeunesse.

Zouves, C. (2004) *A Dream Come True*. Zouves Fertility Center.

Organizations and websites—more resources to inform, inspire and support

ACCESS: Australia's National Infertility Network—www.access.org.au

Australian Donor Conception Network—www.australiandonorconceptionnetwork.org

American Academy of Adoption Attorneys—www.adoptionattorneys.org

American Fertility Association—www.theafa.org

American Society for Reproductive Medicine—www.asrm.org

British Infertility Counselling Network—www.bica.net

Creating a Family—www.creatingafamily.org

Daily Strength—www.dailystrength.org

Donor Conceived Perspectives: Voices from the Offspring—www.donorconceived.blogspot.com

Donor Conception Network (UK)—www.dcnetwork.org

Donor Conception Support Group (Australia)—www.dcsg.org.au

Donor Moms Support Network—www.donormoms.org

Donor Sibling Registry—www.donorsiblingregistry.com

Fertile Action—www.fertileaction.org

Fertile Hope—www.fertilehope.org

Fertility Associates New Zealand—http://fertilityassociates.co.nz

International Council on Infertility Information Dissemination (INCIID)—www.inciid.org

In France—www.pmanonyme.asso.fr

Infertility Answers—www.infertilityanswers.org

Infertility Support Network—www.infertilitynetwork.org

International Donor Offspring Alliance—www.idoalliance.org

International Premature Ovarian Failure Association—www.ipofa.org

Israel Donor Families—http://israelidonorfamilies.org

IVF Friends, Inc.— www.ivffriends.com.au

National Fragile X Foundation (FXPOI)—www.fragilex.org

National Gamete Donation Trust—www.ngdt.co.uk

Parents via Egg Donation—www.pved.org

RESOLVE: The National Infertility Organization—www.resolve.org

Single Mothers by Choice—www.singlemothersbychoice.org

Society for Assisted Reproductive Technology (SART)—www.sart.org

South Western Ontario Donor Conception Network—www.donorconception.com

The Daisy Network—www.daisynetword.org.uk

The Donor Conception Support Group—www.dcsg.org.au

UK Donor Link—www.ukdonorlink.org.uk

REFERENCES

Adams. S. (2012) "Women could delay the menopause indefinitely with ovary transplant." *The Telegraph*, July 4.

The American Society for Reproductive Medicine (ASRM) (2007) "Ethics Committee of the American Society for Reproductive Medicine. Financial compensation for oocyte donors." *Fertility and Sterility 87*, 5, 1001–1004.

Bernstein, A. (1994) *The Flight of the Stork: What Children Think (and When) about Sex and Family Building*. Indianapolis, IN: Perspectives Press.

Bernstein, J. (1996) 'Implementation of Ovum Donor Technology: Start-up Decisions, Challenges and Problems.' In M. Seibel and S.L. Crockin (eds) *Family Building through Egg and Sperm Donation: Medical, Legal, and Ethical Issues*. Burlington, MA: Jones, Bartlett.

Blythe, E. (2009) "Tackling Issues in Cross-Border Care." Available at www.bionews.org.uk/page_38069.asp, accessed on April 11, 2013.

Bohanek, J., Marin, K., Fivush, R. and Duke, M. (2006) "Family Narrative Interaction and Children's Sense of Self." *Family Process 45*, 39-54.

Burstyn, B.S. (2004) "The new underclass." *New Zealand Herald*, February 7.

Cardin, N.B. (1999) *Tears of Sorrow, Seeds of Hope: A Jewish Spiritual Companion for Infertility and Pregnancy Loss*. Woodstock, VT: Jewish Lights Publishing.

Carney, S. (2010) "Unpacking the global human egg trade." *Fast Company*, September 1. Available at www.fastcompany.com/1676895/unpacking-global-human-egg-trade, accessed on December 31, 2012.

Center for Bioethics and Culture (2011) *Eggsploitation* (film). San Ramon, CA: Center for Bioethics and Culture.

Chopra, J. and Weill, C. (1973) *Joyce at 34* (film). Madison, WS: University of Wisconsin.

Cohen, C. (ed.) (1996) *New Ways of Making Babies*. Bloomington, IN: Indiana University Press.

Cooper, S. and Glazer, E. (1994) *Beyond Infertility*. Lanham, MD: Lexington Books.

Cooper, S. and Glazer, E. (1998) *Choosing Assisted Reproduction: Social, Emotional and Ethical Considerations*. Indianapolis, IN: Perspectives Press.

Crockin, S. (2005) "How do you 'adopt' a frozen egg?" *The Boston Globe*, December 4.

Crockin, S. and Jones, H.W. Jr. (2009) *Legal Conceptions: The Evolving Law and Policy of Assisted Reproductive*. Baltimore, MD: Johns Hopkins University Press.

Deech, R. (2003) "Reproductive tourism in Europe: infertility and human rights." *Global Governance 9*, 4, 425–33.

Eaton, L. (2004) "Parenthood is redefined, but custody battles remain ugly." *New York Times*, June 12. Available at www.nytimes.com/2004/06/12/nyregion/12custody.html?pagewanted=all, accessed on December 30, 2012.

Ellender, S. (1998) "Enduring Losses." In E.S. Glazer (ed.) *Experiencing Infertility: Stories to Inform and Inspire*. San Francisco, CA: Jossey Bass.

Glazer, E. (1998) *The Long Awaited Stork*. San Francisco: Jossey-Bass.

Glazer, E. (1998) *Experiencing Infertility: Stories to Inform and Inspire*. San Francisco: Jossey-Bass.

Glazer, E. and Cooper, S. (1985) *Without Child*. Lanham, MD: Lexington Books.

Glazer, E.S. (2002) "A worthy gift, a difficult task." *The Boston Globe*, June 23.

Goldman, E. (2012) Personal conversation with Ellen Sarasohn Glazer.

Golombok, S., Readings, J., Blake, L., Casey, P. *et al.* (2011) "Children conceived by gamete donation: The impact of openness about donor conception on psychological adjustment and parent–child relationships at age 7." *Journal of Family Psychology 25*, 2, 230-239.

Gordon, E. (2011) Personal Interview.

Gurtin-Broadbent, Z. (2012) "Evaluating egg-sharing: new findings on old debates." *BioNews*, April 23, 2012.

Henig, R.M. (2004) *Pandora's Baby: How the First Test Tube Babies Sparked the Reproductive Revolution.* New York, NY: Houghton Mifflin Company.

Indichova, J. (2001) *Inconceivable: A Woman's Triumph over Despair and Statistics.* New York, NY: Broadway Books.

Kalfoglou, A.L. and Geller, G. (2000) "Navigating conflict of interest in *oocyte* donation: an analysis of donors' experiences." *Women's Health Issues 10*, 5, 226–39.

Kirkman, M. (2003a) "Egg and embryo donation and the meaning of motherhood." *Women and Health 38*, 2, 1–18.

Kirkman, M. (2003b) "Parents contributions to the narrative identity of offspring of donor-assisted conception." *Social Science and Medicine 57*, 1, 2229-42.

Kirkman, M. (2004) Personal conversation.

Kramer, W., Schneider, J. and Schultz, N. (2009) "US oocyte donors: a retrospective study of medical and psychosocial issues." *Human Reproduction 24*, 12, 3144–9.

Lazare, A. (2004) former Chancellor of University of Massachusetts Medical School quoted from presentation at Massachusetts General Hospital.

Lehmann-Haupt, R. (2009) *In Her Own Sweet Time: Unexpected Adventures in Finding Love, Commitment, and Motherhood.* New York, NY: Basic Books.

Levine, A.D. (2010a) "The oversight and practice of oocyte donation in the United States, United Kingdom, and Canada." HRC Forum.

Levine, A.D. (2010b) "Self-regulation, compensation, and the ethical recruitment of oocyte donors." *Hasting Center Report 40*, 2, 25–36.

Levine, A. (2011) "The Oversight and Practice of Oocyte Donation in the United States, United Kingdom and Canada." *HEC Forum 23*, 15–30.

Lieber Wilkins, C. "How to Talk with Kids about Their Unique Conception." Available at lafamilybuilding.com, accessed on April 2, 2013.

Lieberman, C.A. and Bufferd, R.K. (1999) *Creating Ceremonies: Innovative Ways to Meet Adoption Challenges.* Phoenix, AZ: Zeig, Tucker and Co.

Lockwood, G. (2012) "Not in Front of the Children." *Bio News 679*, 29 October.

Lorbach, C. (2003) *Experiences of Donor Conception: Parents, Offspring and Donors through the Years.* London: Jessica Kingsley Publishers.

Ludden, J. (2011) "Donor-conceived children seek missing identities." NPR on September 18.

Macklin, R. (1996) "What Is Wrong with Commodification?" In C. Cohen (ed.) *New Ways of Making Babies: The Case of Egg Donation.* Bloomington, IN: Indiana University Press.

Martin, J. (2004) "Court rules sperm donor is not liable for children." *The Seattle Times*, May 7. Available at http://seattletimes.com/html/localnews/2001922232_spermdonor07.html, accessed on December 30, 2012.

Merz, B. (1988) "Clinical Alert Gives Breast Cancer Date, Revises Recommendations." *Jama 260*, 2, 153–154.

Meyer, C. (1997) *The Wandering Uterus: Politics and the Reproductive Rights of Women.* New York, NY: New York University Press.

Montuschi, O. (2012) *Mixed Blessings.* Available at www.dcnetwork.org, accessed on February 25, 2013.

Moorhead, J. (2012) "'I kept thinking, there's a couple out there whose lives I could change.'" *The Guardian*, July 7. Available at www.guardian.co.uk/lifeandstyle/2012/jul/07/infertility-ivf-egg-sperm-donation, accessed on December 31, 2012.

Morell, S. and Morell, P. (2011) *Misconception: One Couple's Journey from Embryo Mix-Up to Miracle Baby*. New York, NY: Simon & Schuster.

New Oxford American Dictionary (2010) New York: Oxford University Press.

Rodrigues, S., Camp-Engelstein, L. and Emanuel, L. (2013) "Fertile Future? Potential Social Implications of Oncofertility." *Journal of Clinical Oncology 31*, 6, 665.

Sandel, M.J. (2004) "The case against perfection: what's wrong with designer children, bionic athletes, and genetic engineering." *The Atlantic Monthly*, April Available at http://jrichardstevens.com/articles/sandel-genetics.pdf, accessed on December 31, 2012.

Schenker, J. (1996) "Religious Views Regarding Gamete Donation." In M. Seibel and S.L. Crockin (eds) *Family Building through Egg and Sperm Donation: Medical, Legal, and Ethical Issues*. Burlington, MA: Jones and Bartlett.

Schneider, J. (2008) "Fatal colon cancer in a young egg donor: a physician mother's call for follow-up and research on the long-term risks of ovarian hyperstimulation." *Fertility and Sterility 90*, 5, 2016.e1–5.

Shidlo, R. (2012) "In Search of Donor Relations and Identity: The Missing Voices of Israel's Children." *Medicine and Law 31*, 641-659.

Shulevitz, J. (2012a) "Why fathers really matter." *New York Times*, September 9.

Shulevitz, J. (2012) "How older parenthood will upend American society: the scary consequences of the grayest generation." *The New Republic*. Available at http://www.newrepublic.com/article/politics/magazine/110861/how-older-parenthood-will-upend-american-society#, accessed on March 27, 2013.

Stack, B.W. (2004) "Egg donor enters battle for custody of triplets." *Pittsburgh Post-Gazette*, July 7. Available at www.post-gazette.com/stories/local/uncategorized/egg-donor-enters-battle-for-custody-of-triplets-542422, accessed on December 30, 2012.

Stone, L. (2004) *Court: Sperm Donor Not Liable for Kids*. Available at www.wnd.com/2004/05/24541, accessed on April 2, 2013.

Smith, S. (2004) Personal conversation with Ellen Sarasohn Glazer.

Stevens, B. (2001) *Offspring* (film). Toronto, ON: Barna Alper Productions.

Tong, R. (1996) "Toward a Feminist Perspective on Gamete Donation and Reception Policies." In C. Cohen (ed.) *New Ways of Making Babies: The Case of Egg Donation*. Bloomington, IN: Indiana University Press.

US Center for Disease Control (2008) *Art Report*. Available at www.cdc.gov/art2008/index.htm, accessed on March 2, 2011.

Whipp, C. (2004) "Why I need to find my father." *Western Daily Press* (UK), January 23.

Wilkins, C.L. (2008) "Entitled to all that parenting has to offer." Available at www.lafamilybuilding.com/pdf/Entitled%20to%20All%20that%20Parenting%20Has%20to%20Offer.pdf, accessed on December 31, 2012.

Zimmerman, E. (2012) "How Cosmo conquered the world." *New York Times Magazine*, August 3. Available at www.nytimes.com/2012/08/05/magazine/how-cosmo-conquered-the-world.html?pagewanted=all, accessed on December 28, 2012.

Subject Index

Author Index